Preface

We live a life for the memories that walk us into what used to be called old age. In the journey through life there are times, a person, an object, and/or a scenario that gives you peace and tranquility. The peace of mind that a person can obtain from a blue sky, a tree for shade, and the memories to think about on a lazy day atmosphere. I have always enjoyed doing activities that were out of my comfort zone. When I would complete one I would tell myself that I was adding to a file cabinet of memories to be reviewed in later years. The tree for shade on that perfect day is something I have enjoyed doing all my adult life. The memories were to be the bonus in my retirement days. Sounds like a plan.

Medical problems interfered with my plans. I have spent over fifty years of my life with no medical problems. Never had a headache or the flu. I could keep going with the idea I was always healthy but it was late in life that I hit a wall. Heat attacks, coma, and death are part of the wall. During this ripple in life's journey I

i

tried to write about some of the things that I encountered during the past three years. A medical problem has four aspects. The problem, the effect on the family, the professionals that will dictate the path of solution, and the patient.

The problem was traumatic but kind in the timing. It hit me and within three weeks the dice were in the air waiting to see the outcome. Quick is kind when measured against a lengthy battle that has health as the prize.

It is during these times the family unit is tested. Each member must look within to muster the determination and courage to face the reality of the problem. My wife and sons showed good quality and resolve.

Fifty years ago I was in the Naval Hospital but the trauma I had was different. I was in a ward and did not see a nurse. All the patients that were able to get out of bed cleaned the ward and then we stood inspection. Then I would collapse into the bed. This time I ended in a mega hospital whose staff had not one slacker.

For the last two plus years I have tried to piece together what had happened. I think I have most the events placed firmly in the time line. I write this as therapy. I have been doing this most of my life. I write what has happened. I then think about it as I read it again. Sentences are added and subtracted. Thoughts are challenged and emotions revealed. Over time my anxiety and questions are answered. I then would throw the paper in the trash. Today technology makes it much easier. I hit the delete key. This activity was taught to me by my mother and reinforced in my college courses. The difference today is the ability to self-publish the writings. It is my hope that it will help someone that believes it cannot get any better. The writing has helped me deal with the future that I might have as a result of my medical problems

I owe so much too so many. I hope their faith, wisdom, and talent were not wasted.

This essay would not be possible without:

my wife - Jo-Anna

my four sons

Robert, Stephen, David, Michael

my brothers

James D and William J

And the prayers of so many

The front cover painting – "The Indian"

The back cover painting – "The Beginning"

were painted by:

Lt Col James D. Nicholson Ret.

Prayer, Luck,

and

a

Beating Heart

By

Robert Nicholson

"Memory is a resource, treat it as one,
it cannot be replaced…but it can be
lost!"

All of us have had that morning when
you wake and can't quite remember
the details to that dream.

"This is where I have lived and revisit
from time to time!!"

Introduction

Was it morning, night, or a dream? My eye lids were barely open and I felt that I have gone ten rounds with a mean gorilla. I lost badly. It was not pain but body exhaustion. It is as if the work out was successful and the body was stressed to the limit. I could barely move. As I laid on the bed, I would guess that I was in a hospital of sorts. That is the only way I could phrase it for I had no idea of where I was at the moment. I attempted to move but could not with the first try. I looked around and saw nurses. The conclusion is that I was in a hospital. I observed as much as I could while nurses were doing many things that I did not understand at the moment. I would observe, analyze, and come up with a conclusion. Using this approach was all I knew and yet I did not know why I knew it. The following impressions and actions may have occurred in a different order but are being written with two important conditions. I believe the order is very close to being correct. The other is to give me an understanding of what was and is happening. How did I get here? Who is the person thinking about all of this? **Who am I?** It was as if a cloud existed around me and I could not make sense of it. I don't know how I know it but I felt if I write, slow the mind, and think small I may remember much more. I have been doing this many times since waking but even at this writing I still struggle with memory and identity.

Observations

I looked around the room using the limited movement of my head. I was lying down on a bed. I was the only person in the room. The room was close to the nurse's station and the nurses were constantly looking in on me as well as monitoring the machines that were hooked into me. There were hoses connected to me throughout my body. On the right side of my waist was a rectangular object a little larger than the palm of my hand. Connected to it was an insulated wire which went into the side of my body. I found out later that the object was a computer of sorts called an LVAD. The wire ran under my ribs to the heart. They bonded the wire under the ribs to the ribs themselves. In the heart was a machine that pushed the blood in one direction. The term LVAD stands for "left ventricle assisting device". Up to this time I have never heard about this device. That means very little at the moment because I can't remember much at all.

The makeup of a person comes from time spent, genetics, and the interactions of the world around them. Which one is more important has always been a debatable subject. My makeup was not known to me at this time because my memory seemed to be a bit weak. I took a deep breath and tried to understand what was happening. I closed my eyes and realized that I am still alive. This was not done with a jump of joy but a conclusion of facts. In the back of my mind was a small idea that at this moment death or life held no difference for me. Live or die, that which follows should be interesting at best and at the least, appreciated. I don't know why I thought this because I don't remember me being in any danger of dying.

There were some other observations that gave rise to some obstacles that will have to be recognized. There was this woman who kept repeating her name and telling me that she was my wife. Every time she would do this I kept thinking maybe I was deaf and that is why she talks so loud. Later I would have young men coming in telling me they were my children. If there were more than one each would say something I could not hear or remember. As this was being done another would be shoving pictures in my face asking me if I remembered something. It seemed the easiest thing to do was to do nothing. They would continue on their own as if they did not need any feedback. In hind sight they were polite and meant well but for some time their relationship to me was not clear. I had some other problems that let me put the family issue on the back burner. I would try to agree with everything they would say while I worked out a more serious problem. I noticed that there was no feeling in my hands or my feet. The feeling was as if they feel asleep but the tingling sensation was not there. I could move the arm at the elbow as well as the leg at the knee. The hands and feet did not obey my mind when I would say silently and then out loud, "move!" They were paralyzed! It is a problem that I will have to contemplate, plan an action, or learn to live with it. Tears or depression were not an option. Why at this time are there no tears. I am sure that I had emotions and yet they are not surfacing as I would expect. I say that as if I knew what to expect when in reality I had no idea of anything. Questions upon questions is

the price of being awake, by myself, and not
understanding why I was laying here.

A Psychiatrist knows all … or so you think!

I was awake. I could now live life to the
fullest I guess. That would be the consensus of
everyone except me. When I was very young I
learned of the Greeks in school. I found two
things to emulate. Their idea of body and mind.
My philosophy of the body and mind was
inspired by Athens and Sparta. This means that
when I am in a hospital bed the Sparta concept of
physical efficiency is in doubt. The Athenian
idea of mind and body was also in a bind. My
memory was almost nonexistent. I should not
say nonexistent. I did have many memories but I
could not line them up. I can remember small
things from my past. But I found out that these
memories are over 50 years old. The amount of
blanks in my memory are evident. Most of what
I would say to those that said they were close to
me must have sounded incoherent. In a very
short time they brought in a psychiatrist to talk
and observe me. My friends and family would
never let this happen if they knew what this man
was about to do to me. After waking from coma

I would drift in and out of a world that I lived in for years. Waking! Wow! I found out I was in a coma for over two months.

I could not tell you the time or the year but the thoughts that I was living with could not have come from this time. It was not a world that I knew but just memories that had no place or time. The world I am looking at today is not part of my immediate thoughts. My thoughts are a mixture of forest, guns, and a couple of friends. These are melting and all I have are memories of death. I would talk to the doctors about me doing things for the government. I would tell them I was not proud of any of the projects I was on yet I could not remember any details. I believe that this is the reason someone brought a psychiatrist in the room to talk to me. This doctor was going to talk to the man with dark thoughts.

The doctor sat in front of me and sincerely told me that whatever I said would be confidential and he just wanted to know me. It took me a while to put everything together.

The story is one that I have pushed deep and it was gone as far as my everyday life. For some reason parts of it were coming back and those parts were not pretty. Without knowing the full story at the time I must have sounded very depressing if not depressed. The doctor made some quick decisions and I was put on suicide watch and a nurse was with me at all times. I did not mind people thinking I was crazy but they bound my hands. These hands had no feeling or motion themselves.

In retrospect, I am curious as to the evaluation that was being done and at the time it was being done. I had just woke from a two month coma and had a few complications getting to this point. After our friendly talk I was restrained in the bed. Being restrained meant that my arms were tied and the hands had large gloves so I couldn't hurt anyone. The problem is that they found me twice out of the ties and gloves. I remembered that 50 years earlier I was trained about techniques that could be used for escapes from bondage.

Why was I stable one minute and a complete change the next? The woman who said she was my wife said I was like Dr Jekyll and Mr. Hyde. This woman did say she saved me earlier with 911 calls. Fate was with me because she saved me once again. This woman was in everyday and saw a dramatic changes in my personality. Upon further investigation she found out the doctor was giving me antipsychotics without any family member's knowledge. My wife immediately put a stop to the medicine and I returned to one personality. I believe that this determined woman saved the person known as Robert, Bob, and or Nick, for better or worse. Would I ever be the person I was is a question that cannot be answered since my memory did not come with a button for reset.

The road from the normal to the surreal

How I got to this point was lost on me for a while. But over time I have begun to remember a little here and there. I don't claim to have a good memory but everyone spend time telling me what happened. A short synopsis of myself at the time this adventure began is in order. Picture a man in his late 60s who is semi-retired. There was one time that I fully retired from all the jobs that I held. They were three of the longest weeks I have experienced. I immediately went back to the local college where I have been employed as an adjunct instructor in the chemistry department. I have taught at the college for over twenty five years. As my memory clears a little, I know that it is one of three jobs I had for twenty plus years and at some point all simultaneous for a number of years.

September 3, 2014

This is a date that made me think about the life I wanted, the one I deserved, the one that I wished, and the one that I lived. Each one is different to some degree. Each one is viewed without the adjectives, good, better, or best. A person must learn to live with their decisions and not with regrets. I lived for the last 50 years with never being sick, no need for medication, and never had a primary doctor. I have never had a headache. When I was younger there were times we would feel a little off and ask mom if we could stay home from school. The "we" stands for two brothers and me. My mother would look close, give us an APC and then tell us we were fine and to go to school. In today's vernacular that would be an aspirin. Needless to say that I and my brothers usually had perfect attendance.

On the day of September 3 I was scheduled to instruct two classes. It was the first day of the semester. During the first class I felt a bit slow so after class I went home to refresh for the second class. It only took me fifteen minutes to go from the college to my house. I expected to enter an empty house. My wife was supposed to be going to the shore for the day but instead she stayed home. I thought I would take advantage of this and asked my wife to make me some scrambled eggs for a late breakfast. For the last 50 plus years I have made my own breakfast. Why on this day did I ask her? I am a person of routine and order. When I make breakfast for myself it is two eggs over easy, two pieces of bacon, orange juice, and two pieces of toast. This is known as my 222 breakfast. Why scrambled eggs? They are the chaos of eggs.

I went downstairs to rest my mind and relax the body. I felt a little weak but a bit of water on my face would give me a fresh start. I went into the bathroom downstairs to wet the face. It is a powder room and the measurement of the vanity to the side wall can't be more than 5 inches greater than the width of my head. After wetting my face I was reaching for a towel

and I lost consciousness. I landed on the floor
between the vanity and the wall. I do not know
how I did not hit either but I landed without a
mark on me. When I woke I went upstairs and
found my wife called 911. I was soaking wet.
The perspiration was the most I have
experienced in a non-stressful situation. I call
this a non-stressful situation because I did not at
that time associate it with anything serious. I
couldn't adjust to the fact that I had fainted. I
have in my life had four known concussions
without any after effect. When I was in college I
fought as an amateur at the civic center. I had a
talent of stopping the opponent's hand with my
head or body. I played football and did many
other activities. While skiing I hit a tree and was
unconscious for a while. How today could I just
faint? My wife heard the noise and came down
to find me on the floor. Hence, the 911 call. It is
the first time she saved my life. When she made
the call they asked her if I was alive. Her answer
was, "I don't know! " I give a number since
there are other times she saved me. I give that a
number but I must also remember fate. (I went
home between classes and that is not normally
done by me. My wife was not supposed to be

home and I did not hit my head on anything
falling into a small divide.) Amazing!

One track, obstinate, or just stupid?

I was upstairs gathering my books and
grabbing my jacket when the EMTs showed at
the door. I must have been a picture. An old
man adjusting his tie while the dress shirt is
soaking wet. The water from my head and neck
was rolling. They want me to sit down and I am
arguing that I have a class to teach and I cannot
be late. I taught at the college for over twenty
plus years and had not been sick. I couldn't let
indigestion keep me away today. I had missed
class due to my parents' funerals. They are both
buried at Arlington Cemetery outside
Washington D.C. I was on the bed as they were
taking my shirt off to get my readings for their
machines. While they were doing this I am not
shutting up. I need to go to work. I couldn't
help the need to fulfill my responsibilities, for
this is the culture I was raised. My body was
exhausted and I could not give any resistance
other than stupid talk which has no rhyme or
reason to it. They had the stretcher and I gave in
since there was no choice. I was alert and

interested in the equipment as we rolled on to the hospital. All of this for indigestion!

Hospital one

We arrived at the hospital with no problems. The wheeling into the hospital begins the adventure into the world of doctors, nurses, pills, appointments, and schedules. They examined me quickly and determined that I needed a stent. While they were putting in the stent they also did an angioblast. I found myself in a bed within a private room with the promise of a quick release from the hospital. I was totally impressed with the modern techniques and the ease at which it was all done. It was told that the indigestion that I had was actually a major heart attack. The doctors said I was very lucky that there was no damage to other systems in my body. I now was ready to leave the hospital. I was in the Navy hospital twice when I was much younger. A time before I met my wife. It was not a pleasant time but I knew when I was getting out and it did not involve a doctor telling me what I wanted to hear rather than the truth.

In this hospital I asked someone when I would be able to leave. I was told an approximate day. When that day came I was ready to leave. I was told that I would not leave until the next day. It was at this point I decided to take matters into my own hands. I got my clothes and decided to sign myself out of the hospital. As I write this it is apparent that I sometimes do not think my decisions through or as complete as I should. As poor my decision, my wife's decision was wise. She had my son bring my older brother up to the hospital to talk sense to me. She knew there are two men I view as the greatest men I have ever known. One is my father and the other is my older brother. My wife's move was done well and after a talk with my brother I went back to my room and declared to the staff I had not signed out and I would like to order dinner. The following day I was discharged and we all went home. It is at this point of the story the words, "And his life went as before and all is well" would come on the screen and everyone would smile at the happy ending.

You could not see a more normal person than me. I was preparing for a return to my classes with my normal scheduling of topics for lectures. I did not yet call the college to say I would be back. After all it had been less than 6 days since my heart attack. I felt refreshed and ready for my next installment of life. This feeling lasted until I was in bed and I couldn't get my complete breath.

Hospital two

I agreed with my wife on this one. She said she was calling 911 and I did not stop her. My status when the EMTs arrived was short on breath and a willingness to go to the hospital. The EMTs were efficient and strong on procedure. I am forever thankful for their strength. On the way to the hospital I died. The description given to me by my wife was as follows: She was in the ambulance and at one point one of the EMTs blocked her vision of me and the equipment. It was at this point she heard the flat line indicator. They proceeded to revive me with their skills. They had to take me to the closest hospital. So my second visit had to be a different hospital, which was closer.

At this hospital they attempted to clear my stent. Apparently my stent was included or known to laymen as clogged. My wife was asked if the stent was approximately ten years old and she had to say it was less than ten days old. While they were observing and working on a plan my condition worsened. It was here that I died for the second time and was resuscitated. The hospital I was in was a Catholic Hospital. It was suggested that my condition was serious enough to consider the last rites. There is always a priest available at this hospital. She asked my brother if she should and he said yes. My wife was told the procedure they were going to try was a 50-50 shot of success. My own opinion is they were being kind.

There are times that something will happen to you and as you think about it in awe you never tell anyone for fear of tainting the rest of a story or your reputation. During the 60s people such as I valued our reputation. In the mid to late sixties I experimented with out of body experiences and transcendental meditation. I wasn't much good at the time but I was not totally inept. Transcendental meditation kept me balanced during many experiences that would have left me in worse shape. My out of body experiences were crude at best but in close proximity to my body I could see or imagine a very blurry silhouette of myself. I mention all this because there was a time at the hospital my other world began encroaching on my present world.

I could not even estimate the time or situation of what was happening. I found myself on a brown coach type seat. On this seat were my two brothers, talking and looking a little on the sad side of the emotional seesaw. I could see other people who were important to me. It felt good they were all here. I just could not relate as to why they were here. I wrote this down but could not attach a tag on it that would make sense to me. Remember I was living in two worlds and this was the beginning of me doubting reality. I did not know in which reality I lived. It has been almost three years and it is only now I am trying to face the events of both realities. While talking to my wife on the order of events it began to fall into place. I believe it was an out of body experience. It correlates to the approximate timing of the last rites and the low point of my health at this juncture. What threw me off was the clarity of the vision and the connectivity to everyone around me. It also answers why no one would answer my questions or laugh at my dry humor. What reinforced this event was when I was talking to my wife and told her the story. She than told me where the seating was in the hospital and told me I described the furniture next to the elevator.

The only procedure they could do was clean as much as they could but in my condition the included stent could not be replaced or cleaned. My condition was not improving so they shipped me over the river to a larger hospital that had the equipment I may need.

Somehow I survived and after a bit of a stay I was declared healthy as possible and I could be discharged. The danger I was facing was the heart racing and accelerating. In order to protect me from this it was requested that I wear a life jacket. This must have been important because they took me into an office and ask very nice if I would wear the jacket. This jacket would protect me from the heart rate rising to a dangerous level. It was designed that if the heart rate was detected above a preset value a shock would be sent through my body. I agreed and we went home with the life jacket.

Who Knew?

For a couple of days I wore this vest everywhere I went. I also wore it to sleep, and to shave. The vest was tight and I thought it was the wrong size. My wife had someone from the company come to the house and see it on me. I was hoping that he would adjust it so I could feel comfortable. The bad news was, it fit the way it was supposed to fit. The vest looked dirty so when I went to shave the next morning I took it off so I wouldn't make it look worse. Over the days the vest didn't have to spark once but in those 10 minutes I should have had it on. Another heart attack and fall. This time into the tub. In all my heart attacks I felt no pain and would joke that I wasn't given a chance to grab my chest and fall to my knees saying something prophetic. Again there was no mark from the fall. When the EMT arrived I was able to walk to the stretcher and was carried to the waiting ambulance. I was getting use to the procedure.

As I was being carried out of the house I saw the woman coming outside from across the cul-de-sac. I had great empathy for her. Her and her husband lost a son a number of years ago. I just cannot imagine the empty space each had to

make whole. She had a problem with her heart
and to protect her she had a pacemaker. I got up
on the stretcher, waved and said everything is
good. Luckily the word good is a comparative
term so I don't have to change it.

Hospital three

I was taken to the nearest hospital. That
meant a return to the second hospital. My
condition was rather poor this time. This was
my third major heart attack and I was told that
any one of them was capable of killing me or
giving permanent damage to my body, mind, or
both. I have died twice in the meantime and I
haven't a clue as to why I am still alive. It is
said that true intelligence is not the formation of
an answer but asking the right question. I only
say this because I have many questions and no
logical answers unless you accept the number 42
as the answer to life. The answer to life
according to the, "Hitch Hiker's Guide to the
Galaxy".

In the course of two to three weeks this was
my third major heart attack. The body was on
the down side and getting worse but my spirit
was, ----------, who am I kidding? I had nothing

inside either. It was a very short time since they saw me so they were familiar with the history and what they saw when I was in before. They didn't waste any time in securing me and coming up with a plan. In order to stabilize me they put a life pump in through my groin. This kept my body in a somewhat stable situation. It was tenuous at best so they arranged a helicopter ride to the next hospital. The interesting part of this is they had to drive me to a nearby high school to get on the helicopter to fly the 10 miles to the roof of another hospital. We made it in about 10 minutes longer than if we had of used an ambulance. This was needed I guess, because of the equipment they carried. I was in my third hospital in the last few weeks but it was number one in the area. I admire the decision to send me to this hospital. I found out later that they decided to do this because if they tried an operation and something went wrong they did not have the next step I would need to survive. You must admire professionals that recognize their limitations when someone else's life depends on it.

Snow white has eaten the apple

Once I was settled in the hospital they began to evaluate me and try to keep me alive while they come up with a plan. My mind is fuzzy at best but this is what I am told happened. My heart was in shambles and the rest of the body was leaning more to death than life. My heart rate was moving higher and the weakened body could not take this for a long period. Whatever was going to happen was put on hold because I was now in a coma. While in the coma I was unaware of this reality. My wife and boys were rallying to make decisions and supporting each other. The immediate family was great and each performed implied tasks. My brothers organized an email chain to many different people and their prayers began. The coma opened up an entire reality to me. It was a place in which I spent a great deal of time. There were the doctors monitoring me and trying to decide how to keep me alive and return me to the world I came from. The question that was coming to everyone's mind was, "will he wake"? In between health problems I talked to all of my boys and each had a job. If they did what I asked the pain to their mother would be minimal.

In the Room of Hope or commonly known as "Last Chance"

There is a room in which the patients that have a short chance of survival are put. In this room the doctors and nurses push to work miracles. The best that I could find is there were a number of us on the most advanced machines available. I can only imagine the pain for my family. It was not that I was in the room and on machines. The problem was every once in a while a box would be brought out of the room. In the box would be a body of a patient that did not make it. My family would have to find out if it was me or not. Death is something my family has only seen in a civilized fashion but even this can contaminate a person. I learned in the late 60s about the effect of death on an individual. I can feel their pain and hope this event would have little lasting effect on them.

My family always had someone present to look and see if the machines indicated that I was still breathing. There were a number of events while I was in the room. My heart was in shambles and they considered a heart transplant. The problem was my body had deteriorated at an alarming rate. The heart transplant was out for the moment. The monitoring machines for the body were to see if the body was operating within parameters needed. These machines gave way to monitoring devices that worked with life aiding machines. I now was not breathing on my own. But I had a machine capable of carrying the load. They had to figure a way to ease the strain on the heart. While I was on the simple machines they did three oblations. This is when they go in and cut scar tissue from the heart. I was now in a coma for over a month and they had to put me on an ecmo machine. This is a machine that moves fluid through the body. The exact operation of the ecmo plasma is not clear to me but I am not concerned about the lack of knowledge. Being on ecmo plasma is one of the last steps. While I was on the plasma they again had to go in and do a fourth oblation.

Why was there no white light?

I had never seen the room of tubes and have never seen the others that were with me. My nickname for the room was the room of tubes. My wife had to spend a lot of time in the room and I accept her explanations. My reference during this time was a bed within the hospital. I was about to have an experience that I see and replay many times. The out of the body experience would raise its head for me again. I could view my body in the bed and then I was somewhere else.

I am standing. But where and on what I cannot say. Then I began walking forward. I stopped and tried to figure out what was happening. When I looked straight ahead and slightly up there was a cloud, maybe. It was like no cloud I have ever seen. It was a cloud with substance. It was not gas but it was not a solid. This unusual cloud had an impression on or in it. The gas looked as a face yet without any definition. I was looking at the impression and I could distinguish a face. It was a face that I could see and yet not quite comprehend. All of this at the same time was weird. From this came a voice that resounded in my head. Yes, I am. My statement was, "you are what?" There was no movement but the voice again resounded in my head. It was a simple reply, "you know who I am". There was no awe or fear as I tried, without success, to see details in the form or in the voice. I was in a reality that had to be explored and must be done at my leisure without the factor of time causing a misconception.

Shortly into our communication I surmised that the one in front of me was of a higher plane of existence. Because I have no other idea of what or who this is I would call the vision "God". I asked why I am here. If I am dying, why isn't there a bright light to guide me? "God" did not address the white light problem but did tell me I was standing there to receive a choice as to what would happen next.   There was a silence while I was behaving poorly. I was trying to touch the substance. It is right in front of me. I reached out and I could not touch it.

The choice

In order to understand the choice, I must tell you about my third son. He is married to a wonderful young lady. The two were married for a while and she became pregnant. Late in the pregnancy there were problems and they lost the little girl. She is on my list of grave sites that I try to visit once every month. It is my attempt to honor them. They are people with no one around to put the flower on the grave. Obviously the young baby always as someone to honor her. Each has great meaning to me. Before my heart problems we were celebrating a new pregnancy for the young couple and waiting for the arrival of a cherished child in the months ahead.

"God" said it very simple. Your daughter will follow one of two paths with the pregnancy. She will have twin girls. If this happens each of the girls will have medical problems that will cause grief in their lives. The twins could have shorter life spans as well. Medical problems was not used but it was implied by my interpretation.

The other path will involve the birth of one girl who will in time be healthy. I wanted to know how the two paths concern my next move. "God" said that I could continue to the next step and I would find it amazing. In the communication now came the concept of death and I noticed that I had no fear of it. I had a genuine interest in the next step. I looked forward to the adventure that would be there. This part gave me contentment because I have grieved for many others I have known. They did not suffer unto death. As King David on his deathbed told his son Solomon, *I am about to go the way of all the earth..."* I have had a good run and was looking forward to the next step.

It was now I found out that if I go on it will be twins. This could cause a lot of pain for the family. If I go back it will be one child and if pain is involved it would only involve me. Sometimes what looks as a choice is nothing more than two ways to say the same thing? I would face "God" three more times.

Dedication, Stubborn, or just hates to lose

It was normal practice to paddle me when my heart rate went above 190. This was done to me many times. My wife told me this became a daily ritual. I would be paddled sometimes twice a day. But to try to resuscitate a person who is dead is something special. One of weeks that I was in the coma I was being monitored by a petite woman who proved her worth as a person of virtue, as well as a fine doctor. I was one lucky person that week. But I have always been lucky. Within a short period of time I flat-lined four times. That in itself is not the remarkable thing. The amazing achievement was an act performed by the young doctor who understood the quality, "perseverance". I believe you could couple this with, "empathy." This amazing person paddled me 27 times in these four flat-line occurrences. I cannot imagine someone paddling me that many times. I was paddled so often that the paddles were left on the bed for quick access. This angel of god refused to give up on me.

When I later had a chance to look back on this heroic act, how could I not give everything I have when I was on my own? I was taught in my family that you have to dig down sometimes to do the right thing. All my life there were three words that were very important to me. This young doctor expanded the meaning of each for me and will forever be thought by me as an inspired angel of mercy showing **"duty, honor, and responsibility"**.

The Coma of 2014

The station is stuck on one picture

I have a poor memory of the beginning but I am told that I was coherent as I laid in the hospital bed. I was losing consciousness and losing the spark that gives me life. The next two months were hell for the family and maybe a few friends. A coma of more than two months does not usually end well. How it is that mine went more than two months and I somehow survived? Of the original group of patients that were in trouble only two made it out of the room alive. And only one of them had no organ damage from the ecmo plasma. Why me? Why am I still alive?

I will tell you what I believe. My older and younger brothers contacted all their friends and gave them the story of my travels to the room of tubes, as I call it. My wife, sons, and people of various churches all got the message out. What message is this that I am talking about? The message is prayer. **The power is prayer!**

I was raised by parents that believed in the message of God but didn't wear it on their sleeve. Church was the Sunday morning schedule. We learned about our religion but more important my mother would take us to other services while telling us about other religions. My parents would say that you have to know your own grass before you can understand the grass on the other side. My parents were too intelligent to tell us there was only one religion and only one way to believe in god. We would discuss the differences and similarities at the dinner table. In my house this was a guilt free area and all could be discussed as long as you were polite. Yes, the dinner table seen in early television before money became the obsession. The Donna Reed Show, Father Knows Best, and even My Three Sons. Family TV in the beginning illustrated the values that mirrored most of America. This is not done today because morals and ethics sometimes interferes with the money train that many people put above contentment.

For the young that are reading this allow me to tell you of a time, and what a time. People thought of ethics, morals, and those that were less fortunate. People of high office and other famous people would give speeches to inform and help. Here is the part that you may not believe. They did not get money for their speeches. They did it to help. It is not as you see today when a politician gives a show and pockets thousands of dollars. People forget those that gave because they can. After President Truman served they had to hold fund raisers to pay his taxes. Today, the millions ....sorry to use politics. This was supposed to be about empathy and truth.

While in the coma I lived another life. The order of my life in the coma may not be in the actual order but it is what I remember. I knew I was in the hospital but not that I was in a coma. As I looked around it did not occur to me that no one talked to me or asked me what I wanted to eat. All I could do was to observe what was around me. I studied the clocks for a while and wondered how in a world where everyone is in a hurry that anyone could get somewhere on time. There was only one hand on the clock. This meant that a twelve hour cycle is the best you could do. I spent days trying to adjust my perception to a twelve hour cycle by looking for day versus night dynamics. I began noticing which was constant compared to which could change. I was on an upper floor and knew that if I wanted to leave for a bit I would have to work on the subtle changes going from the bed to the outside.

The first thing I did was to understand what strength I had left. I would do sit-ups and isometrics which I learned from my high school football coach. Isometrics is the concept of force, effort, without movement. I didn't have the clocks totally figured but I noticed that on the weekends and at night there were openings in their security. It seemed to me that each floor had different colored socks for the patients. I noticed this when patients from other floors would walk by my room. I had to somehow procure multiple colored socks.

I was very busy trying to come up with a plan to get out of the hospital for a walk or just a change of scenery. Confinement is a curse for me and I could not figure out the reason it scared me so much. I could walk quiet and move with grace when I needed. I was able to get out of the bed using very slow motions but had to concentrate very hard. Mental gymnastics are much more tiring than physical movements. I was pushing my mind for everything it had and began using techniques I acquired fifty years earlier. In the sixties I dabbled with transcendental meditation, mind power, and outer body experiences. It has been over fifty years and my mind did not seem that strong but with work and perseverance I was able to move. I picked the night shift on the weekend for a reason. There were fewer nurses and they were tired. I was able to walk by them quietly and they did not notice me. I used the steps by the

doctor's lounge and was able to take a bath robe
and slippers. I was on my way.

Cashing the Check

I found myself on a four lane highway which
I remembered. As a child I would have to cross
it on my way to school. I was in San Diego. It
was a community known as Clermont. The
dichotomy of Clermont and the hospital being
separated by approximately three thousand miles
did not enter my mind. I was familiar with
remote viewing so the logic though sloppy was
accepted. The bank was within walking distance
so I went in to cash a check. I needed one
hundred dollars. I didn't have any checks on me
but I knew I could use one of the bank's checks
after they identified me. I could not tell who I
was dealing with at the bank. The person was
polite and when he gave me a blank check he
said just put your name on it. It was then I
realized that I had a small problem. I did not
know who I was. I didn't know my name or any
personal data about my person. I was almost
ready to panic. Panic was not in my nature. The
situation you find yourself in is because you are
ready for it. I was taught in life as well as the
bible that you sit in the back of the bus and when

appropriate you will be asked to move forward.
Where do I go next? What if I can't get there?
How do I get back to the hospital? Where is the
hospital and what if I am later than I planned?

Sometimes you just need to rest

I began to walk from the bank and when I
lifted my head I found myself facing the
hospital. The car garage was underground but I
saw an access to get in to the car area. I would
pass a security guard if I were to walk directly
into the garage. The questions he might ask
could cause me some trouble because I was
AWOL from the hospital bed. The cement wall
had a small opening. It was very difficult but I
was able to twist through it to the cars. The view
of all the cars. I look and cannot believe it.
There, right there is my car. It stood out among
all others. It was my first new car that I ever
owned. It was a 1989/90 caprice. I drove that
car for 300,000 miles with only three small
replacements under the hood. I thought I lost
this car in 2009 when it was T-boned by a car
speeding in the middle lane while I was crossing
the lanes. His fault, but I thought I lost the car
due to damage. Using logic, I was able to
understand that my family must have had it fixed

to surprise me. It is the only thing that makes sense.

It was in the first row against the wall with cars on three sides. You could see that blue paint against a sea of beige. I got into the driver's seat and put the seat back with the intention of getting some sleep before I attempted the return to the hospital bed. I leaned back and noticed that there was someone sitting in the passenger seat. Whoever it was I could not identify the sex or the face. I felt good that the person had somewhere to sleep instead of the streets. I was also happy that my back seat was large enough to hold someone's belongings. As I leaned back on my car seat I knew that today was good and the adventure interesting. My eyes shut quickly, the sleep was good. When I awoke, I was again in my hospital bed.

The presence in the car

I lay in my bed and questions are appearing in my mind. The questions were actually appearing in my mind! It was as if I was in Time Square looking at the printed word pass. Two of the questions I saw were, where do I go this weekend and can I get back when I don't know how I got back the last time. It was a beautiful evening and the escape was much easier now that I had a path to follow. I walked but could only think about my car. Someone brought it here so when I was discharged I would be able to leave. The idea that one of the family would take me out of here never entered my mind. My initial problem appears to be just the beginning. The questions kept moving across the room. I mean that I could see them. The first of them seemed to be in larger print. That one must have been important. It was who am I? I can't remember many parts of my life while some images I view are memories that I know. I personally buried these memories deep inside. The pain would not affect me because I never let

them into my mind. These memories are mine
and maybe I need to know them but not the
people around me. I need to sort the options
with the problems and see paths of solutions.

I didn't know my way around town yet so
where could I go to meditate? The car was the
only choice. I approached the car and noticed
the same figure in the shot gun seat. I sat behind
the wheel and began to hunt for the mantra. The
mantra was a scene for me. It helped me to
focus and push all the chaos from my mind. I
have been meditating for the last fifty years. My
eyes opened and the passenger was all I could
think about. The passenger didn't move, talk, or
have any distinguishing characteristics. I
couldn't identify the clothes, face, or height. All
of this and it didn't matter. Without saying
anything I felt safe, content, and optimistic. The
feeling I had reminded me of a movie. Spencer
Tracy was an angle protecting a young flyer.

I now had to answer who was I, how much
can I remember, and how close to the present
will be the memories? With this I looked to the
odometer and said, "How can I mentally setup a
flow chart with path, problems, possible
solutions, and consequences with a damaged

memory?" For those that never thought in this progression it probably sounds weird. I was a mathematics/Science major with minors in philosophy and religion. This is the way I always think. Now you may understand my need for meditation.

Memory Lane

While I was meditating the time and location seemed to move. This time I found myself in a back yard pit. The patio was the center and in a Greek style amphitheater the ground rose with beautiful evergreens in just the perfect locations. I found myself seated about three evergreens up the embankment. Whatever was happening looks as if it was done and now we could all leave. I walked down an incline and to the street. This street is in Oceanside, California. A few houses down the street I stopped at a house I recognized. I don't know why but I was walking to the front door of the house. While putting this together in the waken state I would recognize it as the house in Oceanside, California. It is the house before San Diego.

On my way to the door I saw my motorcycle on the grass and a broken one next to it. I went

in and said hello to my older brother. I knew he
would be here. He and my father are the two
greatest men I have had the pleasure of knowing.
We talked a bit and the conversation must
remain with me for a while. After our visit we
stood on the driveway. I wanted to ask him
about the motorcycles. They were identical and
they looked just like mine. As we said goodbye
I got on my cycle and looked around. The sight
amazed me. I could see and recognize all the
people that my brother and my wife would later
tell me about. They were constantly asking
about me and praying for me.   I said hello to
Frank, Al, and Heath. There were so many
living on the same street and I knew them all. I
was told the road was smooth and the weather
good. It was then that Heath said to remember it
all because you would not be here long. Heath is
a friend that I have not thought of in more than
fifty years. He was next to me when he was shot
and lived long enough to say that one day we
would talk again. A true friend is thought of as a
family member. He was a good man and not the
only one I would morn. The past should stay in
the past except for the mellow time when I think
of all. I have spent most of my life thinking of
good people I have met and hoping they had a

good life. For many I visit cemeteries on a frequent basis.

Jim told me where I lived. He said right around the corner. I got on my cycle and rode around the corner. I went in the back through large French doors and I viewed the second level balcony. It was a beautiful home with white curtains flowing in the wind. I was alone in the home and it seemed natural. I went back to my brother and asked him if I lived alone. He said that we learned while young that you must help yourself with faith, tranquility, and peace before you can let anyone in. I thought for a minute and I could only end with, I only wanted a yes or no. I would spend time on numerous adventures. Most were with a woman who could be identified as one of two women in my life. If ever asked which two and of the two which one did I prefer my memory problem will be a little worse than before. This is the best I can do on the identification. Other than me knowing she is my soul mate, I could not truly see the face or height distinctly at any time.

Standing room only

I found myself on a stage giving a speech to a full house. It was at the end and I could only remember the end of a sentence that went, "**and that is my philosophy and reason for my existence**." In the audience was a single woman, known as the love of my life. I would someday like to remember the name she was using. She was brunette and had a number of curves. She might have been my height but I think she was shorter. She took me by the hand and we entered another room that also had a stage. On this stage was a man that resembled a television actor and the girl that held my hand resembled the actor who played his daughter. He and I sat at a table and discussed his daughter and the entire gender as well. I barely understood women, but by the time he finished I realized it was better not knowing anything. At this point I faced a door with her hand in mine and the door opened and there was a well know actor standing there giving me advise about my love. The door proceeded to repeat this another four times with different people telling me the way I was to act, impress, and enjoy her.

In all the discussions I heard some philosophy that helped me enjoy a full dating life and understand a part of my marriage. When you look at problems people encounter a great many of them deal with what my brother and I call the joker in the deck. All the Hollywood types and the John Does around you. With all good intentions sometimes the joker messes everything. The joker is sex. I was very fortunate in many ways. Whether it was my family or a friend, I found the idea that allowed me to enjoy women as equals well before it was law. It does not matter if I was a child, teenager, twenty one, or older the philosophy holds. Sex with the opposites is defined as whatever is comfortable. If holding hands is the limit than that is sex at that time, for the person you are with at the time. The concept of having to bed the date keeps people from enjoying the person they are with. This idea has given me some of the greatest dates and activities. I enjoyed the walk, tennis, roller skating, and many other activities with my date. But sometimes it cut my date short. I never dated anyone just to bed them but some of the girls I dated in college did. These dates were short in time and no second date.

In my alternate reality the girl was a source of belonging. The odd thing is that I couldn't see how tall she was nor did I ever really get a good look at her face. That really does not matter. She fits the description of my wife and maybe others. Like most men, I dated a certain type of person. She and I would go on and have adventures galore. With each new expedition we gained more respect for one another. As time goes on I remember more and more of them.

Never mess with her man

The first event I remembered was very clear. My motorcycle was an air scooter with air intake and exhaust. It was two tone, metallic burgundy and vanilla. I did not ride on the road but above it. Memory of the adventure began to appear. This is the way it happened. I arrived next to a stream and the bike lowers to the ground. I notice a tavern up the hill and decide to have a beer and people watch. People watching was one of my more enjoyable activities.

I go in the tavern and have a seat. I always sit
with the wall to my back and have an
observational plan for exit. I have been doing
this my entire life. I was wearing my motorcycle
clothes as I drank my beer. One of the young
ladies came over and wanted to dance with me. I
said yes and we began to dance. Three
gentlemen took offense to this and pulled the girl
away and turned to face me. Walk outside was
the request. I said I would meet them. I was
exhausted and didn't feel up to this but
sometimes you have to dig deep. We all walked
outside. It was a beautiful evening and the scene
was from a picture. The flowing grass, the
stream, and just across the stream was my
motorcycle. At that moment I noticed my girl
letting her cycle down and turning it off. She
called me over and I turned to the three fellows
and said excuse me for a minute.

When I was close enough to my girl she
asked me to sit at the table. I did but she didn't
walk toward me. She just said," I have this" and
proceeded to walk toward the three guys. I have
heard the description, "like Grant took
Richmond" but I didn't see the video until now.
I was sitting sipping my beer as my partner was

protecting me. Sweet! I leaned back and remembered.

I meant God four times. On the third meeting I was told that my partner would have my back when I couldn't see it coming. It was a year later that I was able to put this together. In the one reality I could sit and have my beer. In this reality I am close to being the person I was before the first heart attack. Whoever I am or how close to the person I was is because my wife had my back. Without her instinctive behavior of stopping the doctor from giving me the antipsychotics the psychiatrist may have created a new person if he continued. I was just getting excited about finding out about the one that was already here.

The Human Mission

In the solar system there were many planets and as with most there were rings around them. The colors were magnificent and each had a clockwise rotation. My partner and I reached the second planet moving toward the inner part of the system. We were being followed and we would have to split apart to complete our mission. Our cycles were fast and easy to maneuver. What was the mission? It was to find and return with a package of great importance. I stayed back and began to lead the enemy away from the area we needed to investigate. I was able to avoid and loose the soldiers that were following us. There was gun fire but as always I lead a charmed life. None of the fire hit me though it was very close.

I returned to the position we agreed upon. I could see in the distance my partner's cycle. When she was close enough I saw she had the package. She reached me and I got a chance to see the package. It was a baby. It was a blue baby. In retrospect this video in my mind represents the meaning of the second meeting of God.

My first meeting I was given a choice to move on or go back. The second meeting was what would happen. With me in the hospital and moving in and out of life, the entire family stayed close. My son's wife was close to the hospital and he also was close. While she was driving she had pain and called my son. My son instructed her to go to the hospital since she was already close. She found the first security officer and told him of the emergency. She was bleeding and in critical condition. The baby was months premature but was delivered and put immediately into an incubator. The baby would be in the hospital for the next three months with many doctor visits after. Today she is a healthy, beautiful, and smart baby. In my youth premature babies didn't have a great chance of surviving. We also called them blue babies.

The fourth visit with the entity that I called God involved the burning bush without consumption of the bush. It was probably me superimposing what I knew of the bible. I cannot reveal the fourth discussion because it has not happened yet. It will happen in 2023. Since this involves known individuals and could be taken as bad or good, it would not be fair to put it into writing.

Decisions, Reality, and Hope

I am not one to remember dates or names. At the moment I don't remember **October 16, 2014**. I say it like this because I was in a coma. My sons and wife will remember it for a longer time. They had to discuss and say yes or no to letting the doctors put a machine in my heart. I didn't have much to say since I was still in a coma.

The device is known as an LVAD. It was during this discussion that everyone seemed to come to terms that I may not come out of the coma. The boys and mother worked well together. I am thankful that when they voted on what should happen there were five of them. This way if the proverbial black marble showed, no one would know who did it and a tie was impossible.

I have always marveled at the amount of pressure the body can take and somehow rebound to a stable situation. It was after the implant of the LVAD that I woke up. The exact time that elapsed I do not know. I was in the coma for two months, give or take. When I say I woke up it may sound as if I rose and everything returned to normal. That is not exactly the story. You are not in a coma for two months, have tests, surgery, and hookups to the most amazing machines and just wake, smile, and go home. This might only happen in the movies. In this world too much has happened. I have to move slowly in this world because at the moment I cannot remember a lot. The other world was so much easier. I am going to try to recreate a sequence of events in my life that may help bring some memories to the forefront. The order will not be chronological but just as it comes to mind. It is my feeling that if it appears it might be important.

A little harder than I remembered

I looked out the large window of the hospital into the hallway. My wife would be here soon and I knew it would be a test of perseverance and will against pessimism. She would be here with the physical therapist to observe me walking. I have always enjoyed pushing the body to the limit as long as I don't sweat too much. This just might be too much. The coma took the muscle structure. The coma took over two months of my life. The coma took some short term memory. The coma took some long term memory. As I thought of this I said to myself, it has taken too much. It is about time I take something back. The thought that came to my mind was the often said sentence from my mother. Things turn out for the best. Maybe they do or maybe they don't but my mother had us so convinced that to this day we just smile and say it was for the best. I was determined to give my best when the show started. It was now show time.

It felt that the paying customers all had good seats. It was now that I would try to recreate the moment that I took my first steps. I will focus on me and the initial try. I can then try to best it in the near future. The coma took my muscle structure. First I had to stand. In the bed I was on my side. My knees were brought up to be level with the waist and I was ready to push myself to a sitting position with my legs over the side. This was a technique I learned in the Naval Hospital fifty years earlier. I have used it my entire life getting in and out of bed. It seemed an eternity and I was tired from just trying to sit up. The physical therapist helped me to stand and shuffle to the walker. I could have done it myself but it was at least 2 to 3 feet away. It was not your normal walker. My hands were not down but at chest level. The walker was tall and looked like a small refrigerator. Without muscle structure I could not hold myself in the upright position with my arms. In my mind I said, "Let us try to give a show to remember!"

I am standing next to this big box with wheels and trying not to just fall due to exhaustion. In my head I hear breathe, just breathe. I raise my foot and attempt to move it forward. It worked!! The back foot is brought even with the forward foot. I don't know if I slid or walked so in my head I walked. They were not full steps but I counted 26 of them in one direction. I was happy. I didn't appear to be jumping but in my head I was jumping and celebrating. I turned around somehow and stood still. I now had to go back. I just wanted to get into my bed and stare at the ceiling. The walk back took a long time and the physical therapist behind me so I wouldn't hit the ground too hard. Fifty two steps and with it the new feeling that not too far in the future I will walk many more!

I could hear them talking. My right foot is dropped. There is no prognosis on recovery from the drop. They were talking negative but I could only hear my voice. I just walked and I felt no pain other than the exhaustion which followed the task. How could I not be feeling good?

Was your optimism earned or just natural?

I have lived my life with the one liners my mother and father would use with us. Most children have heard them during my time. Eat all your food. There are hungry children in other countries that would love to eat that food. Early to bed and early to rise makes you healthy, wealthy, and wise. If you are going to do it, then do it right! All parents should know that well after their deaths the children still hear you. Every time a decision was made I could hear my parents and their sayings. It is times such as this that I hear my mother. Things work out for the best. I always say that even if they didn't she made it seem like it did and in the end that is what made it, "for the best." I thought that I was as pleasant as I could be after I woke from the coma. My wife kindly brought me up to speed. Apparently I was not a good patient and at times made all the other patients look tranquil.

I had just woke and am in the intensive care unit. My hands and feet are paralyzed. I have a memory that works slightly less than my feet and hands. A team of four doctors came in on day and said they wanted to examine my hands and feet. They began to talk about the situation with my hands and feet. They asked me if I could

move them and I said no. They then began
poking me with a long pin. I tried to watch but
couldn't see everything. They said they poked
and I would say I could not feel it. For the feet
the feeling point was at the lower ankle region.
With the hands it was just above the wrist. We
talked and they mumbled something. I never
saw them again. Now what do I do?

The Duke Wins Again

I would lie on my back and try to think of
anything in the past. It seemed that the further
back I thought the better the memory. My feet
were exposed and I would stare at them and
wonder what I would do if they stayed this way?
I looked at the feet and tried to see if the vibrator
on the ankle was working. My memory was
bringing me a picture. It was a man on his
stomach looking at the reflection of his feet. It
then came to me. I couldn't remember the name
of the picture but it was John Wayne doing a
biography of a Navy flier who was paralyzed.
After a long time of watching his feet his big toe
moved a little. That was all he needed to work to
a level he could walk with crutches and braces. I
looked and stressed for a long time and I finally
moved my toe on my right foot. I now knew that

it will work out for the best, with just a lot of
work and luck. My life has always been filled
with both. The Duke was one of the few stars
we saw in California. My father was stationed at
camp Pendleton and John Wayne was filming a
war picture there. Thank you Duke!

Let's Play Ball

What was going to happen to the hands? I
have spent most of my adult life trying to be
mellow and temper free. Coming out of the
coma brought pictures into my mind that I have
tried to forget and bury. These involve the time
line of the late 60s when I did some work for
people representing a government agency. I had
buried this successfully until my three major
heart attacks and the coma. According to my
wife I was not as pleasant with the nurses as I
thought I was when I woke from the coma. This
information will forever lay heavy. These nurses
and their genuine caring had a greater effect on
me than any of the medication I took. The
empathy and professionalism each illuminated to
the patients such as I were as important to the
cure as the doctor's observation and action. I
watched the nurses work hard and still had time
to keep me on schedule despite my wallowing in

self-pity. I can only remember some of it but the parts I can remember don't show me in a good light.

In my life I have tried to stay steady despite the ups and downs of the external pressures. My mental discipline development has allowed me to do this with minimal effect to those around me. The coma took my barriers down for a brief time and exposed to others a side I try not to show. All my jobs have needed a person with no baggage and an empathy for others. The empathy was easy because I was raised around people who believed in it. The baggage was mine and no one else's. I was raised also with the idea that what you did, you have to carry. There is always an etiquette or protocol to how to behave. Each situation requires the correct mental approach before action. I did not do this when I first woke up.

My hands did not respond at first but I kept working them the best I could with my bad attitude. The nurse would give me a ball to squeeze and I would throw it away. I was bound by physical disability and the world was not black and white. I need my organization. I need to know where I belong. I need to know that I would be independent and not a burden to another. That's it! The last one is the most important. Without independence life did not look to appealing.

Transition to the Real World

I was now awake and somewhat alert. I had a wire in my side going from the computer to the heart and another two wires from the computer to two large batteries. Each battery was large, heavy, and they worked. I came into the hospital just under 200 pounds. When I left the hospital I weighed 150 pounds. I had a reserve kit for the LVAD which contained two extra batteries and an extra computer. If for some reason the computer or batteries fail to work I would be in some stress. I always felt that if either failed to work it would slow me but not kill me. This was only my opinion.

The doctors that I dealt with are from the heart failure team at the University of Pennsylvania Hospital. There was not a slouch among them and as always there is one that stands above the others. A patient's opinion sometimes is the guiding light. This man could tell me I was going to die tomorrow and I would thank him. He is the one they would have talk to me when they wanted me to do something. In the evenings sometimes he and I would talk. It was good.

The time is just a few weeks until thanksgiving. The message he is delivering is the request that I go to rehab before I go home. This is a large request in my world. I feel that the situation I am in is the one I will carry to the grave and therefore I should have say in what happens to me now. I may sound like a bastard and maybe I am at times but remember that it is not by birth. I am self-made. Needless to say that with the main man asking me I said yes. Because it is me, I did add a request. I said that I would go as long as two stipulations were understood. One was I would be home for thanksgiving. The other was that the physical therapist be a true DI (drill instructor) and push me as hard as he/she can.

The rehab was not too far from the hospital but the level of nursing was much different. They were understaffed and could not give the individual attention that I received at the hospital. The empathy and skill was the same but the sheer number ratio prohibited individual attention. The physical therapist fulfilled my requirements. Not only were they good but if I left five minutes early they would come and get me later in the day to get back those five minutes. For that I must say thank you.

Introduction to the Rehabilitation Institution

At the rehab center the schedule was set. Meals and normal visitations from the doctor in charge. The physical therapist would take me for two sessions every day that would last about an hour each. They kept track of time so I didn't care how long. I only cared that they would push hard and give me a chance to see what my body can do in return.

I entered the rehab still having a feeding tube in my throat. The person at the hospital that was in charge of my swallowing test was on the border as whether I could have the tube removed before rehab or keep it in a while during rehab. All the nurses that I had at the hospital thought that I passed the test but they do not have the final word. They are the ones that pushed for the test before I was to leave the hospital for rehab.

The tube meant that my food was not solid and real to my senses.

I spend my first hours on the first day trying to get someone in authority to remove this tube or at least give me the attention and tell me how long I have to endure. What happened that night was amazing. I had a coughing spell and this long tube that was called my feeding tube somehow became dislodged. At the end of the coughing I was sitting up in my bed holding the feeding tube in my hand. I was amazed that something that long could come up with just coughing. The doctor on call that night was summoned by the nurse. They both assured me that they will get a doctor in to replace the tube. It was at this point I asked, "Do I have the legal right to refuse the tube?" He then replied," yes." That was that moment. I no longer was dependent on a feeding tube. I told the story to my family. They laughed, but I think they had a hard time believing the story of the cough. They did not swallow my story. (Sorry, had to use it)

Never forget your first time

For two meals I was not allowed to have solid food. I had to be cleared by the top nurse because of the number and size of my previous tracheotomies. When she came I was asked to do a number of small tasks. She would observe my throat while I swallowed and feel my neck. At the end it was determined I could eat what I wanted. I have to give her credit for what she taught me. When I have to swallow the pills I now move them to the back of my tongue and straighten my head. The proper way to swallow. The adventure or the coma could be responsible for the lack of memory of taste. I don't bother trying to figure which. If you were to taste a food for the first time, to experience the flavor, to absorb the juices how would you receive the many tastes and smells for the first time? I had been in the hospital for a while so it did not occur to me I did not remember taste.

My wife called and I told her I could eat regular food. She asked me what I would want. I said, "Burger and fries!" I also said it was to be cooked at home. I knew it was her that walked in but all I could think about was the hamburger. It was in my hand and I spend some time just enjoying the aroma, moisture, and the way it sat the bun. The first bite was not big but large enough to fill one quarter of the mouth. When I was young we were taught this with the number of chews before swallowing. We never had money but enjoyed everything we had. I chewed slow and deliberate as each bite released a sizzle on the tongue. I kept the burger close to my mouth to allow the odor to be inhaled. The smell accounts for the completeness of the taste experience. As I ate the rest of the burger I realized that as good as the others will be, there will never again be a first. I have said and will say many times, "the purpose of life is to gather many good memories to enjoy life at an older age". These are the years I call the ledger years.

Actual compared to Theory

I try to be a realist when I am evaluating myself. How do you handle bad news? This is a question that I would ask myself many times the first night and at least once every day I was in the rehab and beyond. My first day with the DI (physical therapist) I was put through common tests to see my baseline. This would be compared to the scores I should have in order to leave the center. The first thing on the list was to stand on both feet for 6 minutes. I got out of the wheel chair and prepared the mind and body. I said I was ready, she started the stop watch. One and a half minutes later I had to fall into the wheel chair. I was asked to stand on one leg and then the other one. She didn't have to time either since I could not hold balance. I am using the word She but I had two DIs and the other would be called, He. It was apparent that during the coma there was a lot of muscle deterioration. I had no side muscles to allow for balance. My legs were two sticks without shape. I could go on but you get the picture.

After the test I worked on hand coordination, upper body strength, and leg exercises. When I was back in the bed I asked the nurse if I could sit in a chair and I remained there most of the day. I began a slow evaluation of myself and tried to set goals that I think I should attain so I could have a normal life. I had to be honest as I gathered the facts of the here and now. I had three major heart attacks with the last one creating the circumstance of the coma. I was in a coma for two months or more. From the beginning to now I had flat lined six times. One or more was a long enough to result in memory loss, both long and short term. There were tubes between every finger and toe while still utilizing the arms, neck, and groin. I have been hooked to

machines for nearly two months. It began with
machines that just monitor, then machines that
gave life support, and then with these machines
an ecmo plasma was introduced. During this
time four oblations were done to the heart. A
machine was added to the heart to assist with the
flow of blood. When I look down to my right I
see a small computer with wires going to
batteries externally and a wire going into the side
of my body to run the heart machine for flow.
Wow! I can understand how someone could see
this as an ending to their normal life. The
question is, "Would I?"

Inspiration is the View Through the eyes of another

After breakfast I had another session with my
physical therapist. I started with moving rings
from post to post and finished with squishing
rubber balls. During my leg exercises I sat a
couple chairs from an elderly woman. She was
old enough to be a grandmother of more than one
grandchild. She was doing some movement with
her legs and had an expression of determination.
I saw a person that didn't complain but worked
hard to reach her goal. She just had both knees
replaced. Next to her was a young man adjusting

a prosthetic leg to prepare for his session. Story upon story was seen around the room from young to old. With a bit of sentimental thought and fear of embarrassment I knew that the optimistic part of me will again triumph. From that point to today as I write this that woman of small statute but great determination is an influence on my outlook. Before I left the rehab I was able to talk to her and tell her of the inspiration she gave me in a time of need. It would have been nice to meet her grandchildren and tell them about her. You see, she was in her 80's.

It is now time to get to work

During my working years I have had jobs involving administration to the worker bee. When I say the working years I mean the years before my main retirement. In my world I always needed to know the rules, expectations, and all the external pressures. I arranged to have the boss come and see me so I could understand the regulations that I had to work within. Every person should know their limitations and then decide whether you stay within or breakout. It is easier to shape your plans than complain about something that cannot be altered. I currently was not allowed out of my bed and room unless I was accompanied by someone and I had to be in a wheel chair. Within the next four days I contacted the person that could change my designation. This was the physical therapist with the resident doctor. With a little work and as much logic that I could muster I was able to get cane status and independent walks. This was done with them knowing my time limitations and a lot of promises from me. Now I had to push and push hard.

I was reminded later of a story I hope I remembered on my own. My son Dave had just broken his femur while boarding behind a boat. Luckily there was an EMT on the boat and he survived to be operated on. They put a titanium rod in his leg and when he left they gave him some crutches. For the next several weeks I would drive him to classes that he was taking so he would be better prepared for his next job. The second day I had him in the car I drove to the store. I had him go in with me. I took him to the canes and said if you can use crutches than a cane will do. He gave me a look like I did not understand pain. I have seen and know what happens to a person who gives in to the situation when they want to be elsewhere. I showed him how to use the cane and he did the rest. In a short time he mastered the cane. Everywhere I drove him I would park far from where we wanted to go and we would walk the rest of the way. In the end he walked well and finished the classes. I am proud of him. I drove him to an interview for the job he has today. I should say that today he has a bachelor degree achieved through his dogged determination. Things have a way of turning out for the best. An example of courage, determination, and he is my son. I have three more interesting stories and by coincidence, I have three more sons. All have shown qualities that I would like to see in everyone I choose to meet a second time.

Be careful, your wish may be granted

It is sobering. I sit in the room and look around trying to put everything in some type of perception. I am in a respected rehabilitation center recommended by a marvelous hospital. I see a walker, wheel chair, and a cane. The wheel chair represented to me complete failure. If you can't go further than the wheel chair is respectable. I also see a walker, which means I cannot stop with the chair. I tried using the walker in the room and realized that if I can walk I should be using a cane. From that point on I would use only the cane unless the therapist said otherwise. Three days before I wanted to leave I had a chance to sit and talk with the top person. She and I sat and talked for a while. At the end we decided that I could go home two days before thanksgiving, which was one day earlier than I wanted originally. Before I could go home I had to take the entrance test again to see if I passed the minimum requirements. I surpassed every one of the activities required. The walking and related tasks were not a problem. The DIs did their job. The hardest of the tasks was the walking up four steps, turning around, and coming down the four steps. I had almost no muscles in the legs which means total concentration and deliberate motion. I did it! A side note should be remembered. I asked the physical therapist to be hard, cruel (if needed), and persistent. They were everything I requested. On the last day the DI came by after dinner. I looked at him and he gave me the look. He did this a number of times during my stay. He said grab your cane. You owe me 12 minutes for the day. I got out of bed and we went to the room to work. A simple thank you is not enough but it is all I had.

I was finally going home. I was sitting in the passenger seat while my wife was driving. We turned the corner and we were finally pulling into the driveway to my house. My eyes were almost tearing as I sat and viewed the beautiful sight. I smiled and realized I did not recognize it at all. I then realized that the amount of lost memory is larger than I thought and I am not sure of its limits. I therefore must keep much to myself. People treat me different now. Just imagine if they knew the amount of life I have forgotten.

If the water seems cold you just adjust

Thanksgiving and the house is full. I sit downstairs on the sofa and don't dare go upstairs. When I get up, move in any direction, or just try to adjust I must be aware of the computer attached to my body. The computer is controlling a device called a left ventricle assist device. The call letters are, "LVAD."   It is on my right side with a wire going into my body running under the rib cage to the heart. There is an adhesive attaching the wire to my ribs. On the other side of the computer is another wire that can be connected to two batteries. The batteries can run the system for about 12 hours before having to be recharged. Each of the two batteries have dimensions of approximately 9in x 2in. They are quite heavy or seem so after trying to hold them for the time you are walking. I would estimate the weight to be about 5 lbs total for the batteries. It was not the weight but the awkwardness of them as you tried to maneuver. This was the second generation of the LVAD. The first was large and had to be pushed on wheels. People would live at the hospital waiting for a heart transplant. The hospital had two floors for them to live on while they waited to see if they lived or died. Heart transplants were not common and the chance of a normal life was in doubt.

I never minded hard work but I know I needed a plan or at least an idea. To do this I needed an organized situation that I understood and could work within. While I was in the hospital I heard of a vest that was made for the LVAD. My wife and son looked on the internet and found the website. They estimated my measurements and immediately ordered a vest.

It would allow me to move without the cumbersome feeling of the equipment that I needed. The vest was heaven sent. It had a pouch for the computer and a pocket on each side to accommodate the batteries. I could now move without carrying the batteries and computer.

Sleeping was something I had to get used to doing with my new equipment. I didn't wear the vest while sleeping. The computer stayed at my side since the wire connected to it went into my body and even at night the computer must keep operating. The batteries that run the computer had to be recharged at night. I would attach a different wire to the computer at night so I could plug into a socket for power. My radius of movement during this time amounted to 20 feet. My bathroom is over 40 feet away. Next to my bed my wife put my walker in the open position. At night I would be able to stand and go in the plastic jug as I did in the hospital. My modesty never left me so at night I had two problems. The first was getting out of bed with computer and wires. The second was urinating without making noise. In time I managed both without waking my wife. Or she was just faking it.

I was getting better with the equipment. As time went on I dropped the computer less. The tug of the wire on the body when this would drop is always remembered.

I had another problem that I had to address immediately. My right foot was said to be dropped. When I first stood in front of a mirror I tried to see how much it was dropped. I could not measure it but the drop could be seen. The two questions that entered my mind were, do I have to alter my walk and is this a permanent condition? The first day in the house I saw the answer to the first concern. I was entering the bedroom when my toe hit the rug and I had no way to keep myself from falling forward. Two months in a coma left me with no muscle structure so when my arms went forward to cushion my fall they had no effect. I could only turn my head and hope I didn't hit anything. When I was on the floor I looked forward and saw I missed the glass door on the cabinet by at least 6 inches. The next problem had now just appeared. I could not push up with my arms to right myself. I had to crawl on my stomach to the chest by the bed and pull myself upright. As

I stood there I realized I was winded and grasping for breath.

Every man should know his limitations so he knows how to push them. More important is the ability to stay within so you can relax a little. I was starting to dream up a plan that I would utilize and it would be extra to whatever I am told to do.

There is always schooling and a lesson to be learned

At home I was entitled to have a nurse visit me twice a week and a physical therapist would visit twice a week. I forget how many weeks I was entitled to because on the initial visit from both I heard the same thing. When you read my medical file it would present for you a picture that did not actually reflect reality. The factors age, heart attacks, coma, LVAD, flat lining multiple times, and nerve damage (dropped foot) would give a picture of the patient.

On each first appointment to get our schedule set they would come in the house and see me sitting in a recliner. They expected someone that was not mobile and not as healthy looking as I was. Each one said that I wasn't as bad as the file and the office indicated. We agreed that six weeks would be sufficient. I admired their honesty and we immediately got to work. The nurse really could not do much other than readings that had to be recorded. My wife was trained at the hospital to change my bandage around the wire every day in a sterilized environment. I took all normal readings that were recorded every day with equipment the hospital gave me.

My physical therapist would explain the appropriate exercises and then we would do three sets. She was the one that gave me a few exercises for my dropped foot. She showed me how to use the stretch band to try to give the foot structure strength. The two of them were always on time and never missed a session. That is important to a patient that truly wants improvement and is willing to push the envelope. Ever since my 20s I have woken at approximately 3:00 am and then went back to sleep. I now used this time every night to work both of my feet with exercises taught to me. Three months later it was noted that the foot was no longer dropped. The big toe was dropped a little which I again would trip on the rug only

this time it was downstairs. I missed the brick
fireplace by at least a foot.

There is always another frontier

From the downstairs to the upstairs there were
6 steps to the front door and another 6 steps to
the other floor. I live in a bi-level. You need
information before an intelligent decision can be
made. I stood at the bottom of the two sets of
steps. I figured that if there were a problem I
should be going up to limit the distance if I fall.
I think I looked at it for 5 minutes. I was not in a
hurry and I mentally figured where on the hand
rail I would place my hand. I would try the first
time walking as I used to with one foot per step.
I took the first step and felt weakness. The
second step gave concern. The third step showed
me the lack of arm strength that should have
pulled me up with help from the legs. The rest
of the way I put one foot on the step and then the
second foot on the same step. Then I did the
next the same way. I now knew what I had to
do. There are six steps per unit so I set the
number six as the times I had to go up and then

down the two units of steps. Each time I did it I would start with a different foot. First time up the twelve steps I would start with the right foot and the second time I would start with the left foot. On each step I would stand straight and go to the next. I used the cane for each step. Each time I did one the pride of doing it, the disappointment of weakness in the legs, and the determination of pushing forward showed. I would look up at the end and say, "God! Life is beautiful." That expression is always followed by saying, "One more day in the ledger, thank you."

It sounds as though I know what I am doing but it could be I am just stubborn. How do you know if the word should be persistence or stubborn. It is all about point of view. You know, it is lifting your right arm and in the mirror it is the left arm that is raised. In my time they used to say walk in someone's boots before you judge.

I would sit downstairs on a sofa watching television and the cable would go out. I knew I had to disconnect the connection and reconnect to start the television. I am alone so I can try a few things without anyone giving me their

opinion. I slowly got on my stomach to stretch
out to work the cable connection. The cable box
is on the bottom shelf in the back of the
television stand. Without arm strength it took a
while to loosen and then tighten the connection.
I did it and felt good about it. Now I put my
head on the rug and rested. I have to be careful
when I do things because I am on strong blood
thinners. With the help of the LVAD it lets the
blood flow easier though my heart. I tried
pushing with my arms but I noticed no
movement. I now had to turn my body and
crawl on my stomach to the sofa. I would get
memories of doing this over fifty years ago. At
that time I again did it carefully. I then slowly
crawled up the sofa and sat down. The
exhaustion was apparent as well as the slight
smile for doing it.

I had to uncover the mirrors on time

I had no strength so I couldn't yet take the
dog for a walk. Walking too far from my house
was not an option at this time. It was only three
weeks earlier I had begun to learn how to walk.
When I woke from the coma I was able to walk
26 steps from my room leaning on a tall walker
and the 26 steps back. I had an idea which I did

not tell my wife until I tried it. I will walk around the caudal sac and never leave sight of my house. It seemed safe since I had good neighbors who would pick me up if I fell. The first time I tried this I made sure I was the only one home. So much for the neighbors picking me up immediately. I will push hard. I am alone because I am tired of everyone treating me as I would break if I sweat. Standing at the top of my steps in the house I am working every possible scenario and how I would react. I am now ready for the inaugural walk. Something like this would set my mental state for recovery so I go slow and deliberate. Hand rail, cane, pace, and care were words rattling in the head and this was just to get to the door.

I stepped out of the doorway and stood in my three point stance. Two feet, one cane, and the riddle of the Sphinx. I had to remember that my right foot was dropped. I have been working hard on the foot so It wasn't dropped much but enough that I had to constantly think, up with my foot and then forward. At this juncture I was not paralyzed but I had no feeling on the top of my feet, the little finger on my right hand, and no feeling on the top of my left thigh where they

had to cut the muscle and move it a little. There
was a slight down slope going away from me. I
aimed for the sidewalk. I began with small steps
and a smile. In my head I would see the words,
bad foot and cane then the strong foot. Why the
smile? There were many reasons but three came
to mind. A chill to the air, clouds in the sky, and
the beginning of my independence. That was
number one. The second would be the picture in
my head of the comedians of my time imitating
an old man trying to get from point A to point B
with many very small steps. The third was a
habit begun young and used all my life in
stressful situations. It would keep me calm
while I could find a solution. It was the slight
smile I would have when everything seemed to
go against me. The smile meant to me that the
problems might be large but I will continue to
push to a solution.

I wander with my mind because it allows me
to connect my past with my present knowing the
effect on my future. My mother made sure that I
and my brothers knew not only our religion but
also many others. One of the religions is the
Jewish religion. Yes the word Jewish is not only
religion but also of a people. Many Jews have a

ceremony known as sitting Shiva. In many of these homes when someone dies mirrors would be covered. It was very important that the mirror is uncovered before the year is complete. This would signify the new beginning. I hope I remembered everything correctly. I have worked for and with Jews and have a great respect for them. When I began the initial walk I had in my mind that the cloth must be removed before the year is completed and I need to know that this is a new beginning.

The Walks of the Circle

It is only a caudal-de-sac. The feeling was the same as I had the first time I sat in a ski chair moving to the top of a mountain. It is only a mountain. My pace was normally 33 inches. Today it could not be more than 24 inches or less. Again and again I would recite, bad leg and cane then the strong leg. I always did talk to myself but today it seemed like a crowd betting would I make it or would I fall? After all these years our sidewalks are not flat. I found this immediately. My toe hit the cement and my balance was upset. I fell but I fell how I had planned. I threw my weight toward the grass and the lawn cushioned my fall. Now would my plan to get up work. It was at this point I yelled at myself for not trying the maneuver before the walk. I purposely tried my initial walk knowing no one was home in the caudal-de-sac. Independence must be mine or at least in my mind.

I am on my side on the grass of a neighbor. I rolled onto my stomach clenching my cane. The lack of strength in my arms would not allow me to pull myself to my knees going toward my cane. The cane had to be placed close to my shoulders in order to push on it causing the body to go backward raising the torso a bit. This technique almost worked. I found that at one point I had to twist the body so I could push at a different angle to get to my knees. Once I was on my knees I looked up and said thank you but I have to rest a minute. The next part is a bit harder. You have to use your cane to stand but if your angle and timing are off you will fall. It is also important to know if you emphasize the arms or the legs. Falling does let you try something else but I was very tired so I needed to do this the first time. After the small rest the strong cane allowed me to again stand in my three point stance.

As I stood there the smile was larger followed with a laugh and settled into determination. I looked at my house on the other side and looked to the corner I was trying to get to in my walk. Naturally I turned right and made it to the corner. I looked around and it was only me and the world. I had to imagine the Rocky music as I yelled out at the top of my voice. I said, **"World, look at me!"** I then looked at my house and needed to set my mind for the walk back. I rested and walked, rested and walked, and rested and walked. It seemed as if the house was moving away from me but I made it to the front door. The body was tired but the energy of success was present. Reality snuck in and I just wanted to sit in a comfortable chair. I entered the house and for a second I said up or down. I laughed a bit because I knew the only option was down. I was exhausted. I made it and closed my eyes and that tranquility. Because I knew that I did it. Now I had to push it.

Repetition

This is something I have been doing most of my life. Structure and organization is my basis, my need. My days may look different but the basics were redounded. Every morning was a walk, every afternoon a walk, and every evening a walk. Every evening my wife would change my bandage where the wire entered my body. It seemed like a lot of trips to the hospital for tests and many trips to the laboratory for blood tests. But for the first time in my life I was living on the honor roll. This would be interrupted after about six weeks.

Who can ever forget their first?

I often look into my magic mirror. Everyone has one. When you look around while you are out and see the plaid shirt with stripe pants. He looked good in his mirror. The woman that hides her face with a lot of makeup looks good in her mirror. You see why I look into mine. I see the wire entering the body, next to me are two large batteries with a computer, and the zipper going from the mid chest to just below the ribs. All I can do is say that I don't look that bad, considering. This was one of the times that my view was true, I think.

This was the first time I tried to look objectively and not emotionally. First times are unusual events. The emotion of the moment overrides the inadequacies of the act. I learned to walk! I can learn more! Along with my thinking of this traumatic event I got to experience another one. You have to wait approximately six weeks after they cut your chest open before you are allowed to drive. Since I got out of the hospital my wife, with a little help from my sons, drove me everywhere. Now I was getting behind the wheel. The first drive was to my brother's house. I had a problem within the first ten minutes. My arms had no muscle structure. My hands start at 9 and 3 but quickly turned to 7 and 5. The first time I had to stop on the road I found the weakness in the legs. I barely stopped in time. This was very disappointing to me because I spent 30 minutes practicing in a vacant lot with my son as the passenger. My entire life or at least what I can remember, I have always been able to adapt. This was no different. With great thought of what I should do and the patience to practice I was able to drive efficiently. The smile, tranquil feeling, and feeling of accomplishment were all present. Again, as always, I said thank you.

I could now drive myself to rehabilitation three times a week. I could now drive to the labs for my blood tests. The time long ago when I learned how to drive was different then today. A young man and a lone highway spelled happiness and tranquility. In a car it was just you and the world. What a feeling. Today I began my journey to independence!

The road looks straight for the rest of my life

I was once again content and at peace with my current life. Since I was a pup part of my prayers would be to find contentment in life. Even as a child I knew that contentment and happiness are not the same but they can be found together. The LVAD does complicate my daily routine but I can adapt. You still have to watch for problems with the equipment. I have four extra batteries and rotate them every morning after I unplug from the outlet. The computer has given me problems twice.

The first time I had a problem with it brings a smile to me every time I think of it. I was lying on the bed watching my wife prepare the sterile situation needed to change my bandage. I heard a beeping and asked my wife if she heard it. She said yes. The sound meant that the computer was not functioning. My wife did great getting my extra computer from the case. She showed patience and a calmness that was followed with confidence. It was then that she tried to undo the connection to the computer I was wearing. It would not come off. The look on her face was priceless. I knew I couldn't smile so I sat up and asked for the computer. She gave it to me and it did take some time but both wire connections came off and the new ones were put on. My wife was a warrior and completed the bandage before sitting down and taking twenty minutes to collect her wits. She immediately called the hospital and they said they would mail one out. She said no. We got into the car late at night and went to the hospital to exchange the computer for one that worked. What could I say? If this one went she didn't want me to struggle. I don't think I would die but it was not tested tonight. The second time it went was not traumatic, especially after the first time experience.

How long can you drive that old car?

I had to go to hospital quite often for testing, checking, and assurance from the heart failure team. The head doctor would talk to me about my activities and you could see that he was trying to assess my feelings as well as my physical status. It was often when my wife was not present I would ask him my personnel questions. The two that I would ask often were important for my future. I have a family that gave a lot while I was indisposed. I owe each.

I needed to know if the LVAD was a destination. In my research I found that it was originally a bridge used to get you to the heart transplant. The heart transplant is not used for the patient that cannot qualify due to the type of illness or **age**. The answer was yes. I than asked how long can I expect to live using the LVAD. The answer was given to me as an average. He said between 10 and 12 years can be expected. I could handle this because I know an average is taken from numbers under and numbers that are over the averages.

Life is beautiful and I have always viewed it this way. I was ready to live my one year or my twenty years. Because I always had one sentence in my head that I truly meant. I have had a good run!

Life turns with every decision

My life is now set and I would learn, push, and adjust. Using these as virtues I felt my situation was going to be fine. Everyone knows that if you have a plan there may be something that could disrupt it. On one of my visits the doctor asked me if I have ever thought about a heart transplant. This is **The Doctor**. He could tell me I was going to die and I would thank him. This is the only thing I can say about him and I do it frequently. I thought I was too old. I was a person that smoked for over 45 years. I asked him why me? I thought I was too old. If I were to say yes what is the procedure? He said that I would have to be interviewed by the heart transplant team first. The interview would be about 5 hours with individual professionals from the team. Their questions can be personal, about your health and the tests that I would have to go through. They would tell me about the procedures before the transplant can be approved. These required procedures would verify if I was a viable candidate. Everything would be covered during the interviews and that would include the financial aspect. I thanked him and said that I would give it serious thought.

What should I do? I am semiretired and have done a lot. My life had a quiet meaning. I have lived my life accepting people for who they are and have not physically hurt anyone (if you ignore three years in the late sixties). I have always been more adept as a lone individual than as a societal person. I was always curious about this behavior.

It was answered on day with a discussion with my older brother. One of our shirt tail relatives did a little research on our family background. Many generations before us, our ancestors, moved from the east toward the west. They settled in the wild and were content. As more people came others would move with them to what would become a town. My relatives did not go with them and became known as, "Deep Woods People." When he was done reading to me we both looked at each other and laughed. It explained a lot and gave us an understanding that we were not unusual but just being us.

Heart or Machine

There is an advantage to keeping the LVAD and foregoing the heart transplant. I am becoming familiar with the machine. The daily bandage changes, adjusting the vest every morning, and the bulge at the waist are beginning to become routine. The medication is tough to get used to because I have never taken medicine on a steady basis. The amount of bruising on the body is mostly covered except for the hands. Blood thinners are a bit rough on the body but essential for the machine to move the blood. I am constantly with the cane and am pretty good with it. With the LVAD I know that I have at least 5 to 10 years to help and enjoy my family.

A heart transplant is a marvel that I thought would never happen in my lifetime, let alone to me. If I say yes to this procedure it will begin the movement of a domino. You have seen dominos set up so as one falls it will cause another to fall and so on. I would sit alone at night and think of the dominos. I would be one of their oldest transplants at this hospital. If the interview goes well I would have to have a battery of tests. If anyone of these tests proved serious then I would not be eligible for the transplant. It would mean many more trips to the hospital than I am already doing. The tension and pressure would increase on my family. My families' hopes and disappointments would move as a roller coaster. For most of my life I have worked many jobs and long hours. My family was the reason I would give myself. This last part is taken from what I can find out about myself. The coma or heart attacks have taken their toll on my memory.

The operation means more pressure and shock to a body that has had three major heart attacks. Each one should have killed me. Officially died six times. Four times they went into the heart to cut scar tissue. I was cut open and a machine was placed in the heart. I barely have muscle structure due to laying for over two months in the coma. There is no assurance that I would get off the operating table. I have lost a lot of memory but I have a lot left. I am physically able to get around. Another operation could leave me in a condition that would require someone to take care of me permanently. In my world this is a worst case scenario. My individual independence is crucial to my being who I am. I understand that I have family obligations but I choose this life. That is different than having to be tied down physically and rely on someone else because you must.

A new heart means a new conditioning of the body. It could mean more visits to the hospital. It could also mean a shorter rest of my life than the LVAD would give me. I realize that this is my decision and mine alone. I use my wife as a wall and ask about different scenarios so I can hear myself out loud. I can also gage her response. Hearing yourself out loud brings in the ears and slows the mind so you can evaluate better. A technique that was taught to me while I was training in my youth.

The real question comes to the choice and the gamble. Would I be more help to my family in the immediate or would I be more help to them further down the road. I myself can handle most anything. I know I could not handle my family watching me die. I look into my magic mirror. What I really see would take much more magic than the mirror can find. There is no muscle structure and basically just loose skin with bone under it. I look at sad sack in the mirror looking back at me and just smile, then laugh a little. This would be something!

Try the Ignition One More Time

I told my wife I was going to do the process needed to get a heart transplant. This was my way of saying that I may not qualify but it won't be because I was lazy or did not give it 100 percent on my part.

The interview was the first step. We went to the hospital in the morning and didn't leave until dinner time. There were approximately five people that came into the room separately. Each would spend about an hour talking about their specialty. I believe each had something in common. As they talked with us I believe they were evaluating if I would go the distance at full speed. We were introduced to the effect it would have on the family. The cost and ways to finance along with programs available were discussed. All the tests that would be done and if one of them was off by much I would be disqualified. My smoking was constantly brought up and I would be meeting with a doctor who was a professional the treatment of addiction. There was no final decision but just an," Atta boy, we will start the testing."

With each test the pressure increases

The battery of tests began with a colonoscopy. The day before the test I got the liquid mixtures that I had to take to clean the system. I always found it fascinating that people attempt to cover something if they themselves feel it is uncomfortable. Everyone kept asking me what flavor I want as if that would make everything bearable. In my small world you have two choices. You either do it or you don't and no amount of flavor will change that. I said give me the unflavored one so I could emotionally understand each step. After all, this was my first colonoscopy.

When it was completed they found two nodules and had to do a biopsy. I was not bothered by this because I knew my run has been good and if the trail to a new heart stopped here I could understand. It bothered me how it was effecting my wife and family. It seemed they were more emotional than I. The biopsy was negative and I could look forward to the next test.

And I was trying to grow it back

One of the tests was a skin observation. I was checked all over and felt pretty good since no one gave me any bad news. I was sitting in a fancy chair you find in a dentist office. A young female doctor came in and began sanding my head. Yes, I mean sanding my head. I could feel

the grinder and imagine what they were doing
from the vibration. I had skin cancer on my
forehead and on my ear. All of these tests were
to see if everything functions as it should but
there is one thing that would cause an immediate
delay in the transplant schedule. That is the
discovery of cancer. Again the angel on my
shoulder did the dance. The cancer was a type
that is isolated and did not spread any further.
The surgery she did is called moss surgery and
she was good. A few visits, a changing of
bloody bandages, and a little skin graphing I was
almost brand new. At home I would look into
my magic mirror and see the image of the
moment. I had a bandage behind the one ear
where skin was taken for graphing. Very high
on my forehead, where hair was seen during my
youth, was skin of a different color and looked as
it would take time to heal. I was told to schedule
the next test.

Who Knew

Our rides to the hospital were frequent and
the tests were many. The last test was one that
fascinated me. This one was my lungs. I was
raised with many protocols but basically two
rules. Do not lie or steal. I can count on one

hand and have fingers left the times I have purposely lied. We do not count the times I was being polite and not going to hurt anyone's feelings. Going to this test I lied. I lied in the sense of trying to see a result. I got this idea from a scenario of my mother talking to a good friend. This woman was normally very gentle but today she was talking about the Jews in a negative manner. When the woman stopped talking to breathe my mother gently said to her that her grandmother was Jewish. In my family we go out of our way never to embarrass anyone. But more important to us is not to degrade any ethnic or religious group. The woman became very apologetic and looked shaken. It was then my mother said she was kidding but knew she got her point across.

When I was asked about my smoking I said I have never smoked. The technician proceeded with the test. I was placed in an isolated container with a mouth piece and instructed when and how to breathe. I was told at the end of the test that my lungs were clear. Who knew? I did this because I wanted an unbiased observation. I read a report out of England that some smokers can smoke as much as two packs a day and have no effect on their lungs. That does not mean it won't affect some other part of the body. My father had lung cancer. I don't know if it was from cigarettes or the three wars he fought, or the collapsed lung he suffered on the pacific island when a bomb went off.

The Cure would work but you don't have the right sickness

My last test was a discussion. You have to be free of nicotine in your system for approximately six months. If you are a smoker you must be free of the nicotine and have not smoked. The doctor we were meeting with is an expert in freeing people of tobacco habits. He was a common man of great intelligence. We talked. I presented him with a unique problem. I smoked for many years and normally would use his advice to stop.

After my third major heart attack I was in a coma. During this time many things were done to me as well as many different liquids put into my body. No one in the room offered me a cigarette. After a coma of approximately two months and a hospital stay followed with a two week rehabilitation stay I was clear of nicotine.

Knowing where I came from and how I was raised I did not crave nor want a cigarette. This was my type of doctor. He was interested in me and not the "me" in a medical book. We talked and we both listened. He said his cure would have worked but at the moment I did not have the sickness. He made it a point to say that habits are there for a reason and if the reason is still there I may need him later. I understood and shook his hand.

Many things are out of your control

I was told we would receive a call from the heart transplant team. The team has two people that work the logistics for the patients. These logistics include many different activities. The ones that directly concern me were the following. Would they accept me? If they do what are some of their actions that would affect me? How does it all work?

There was an A list and a B list. Which one would I be on? Where would I be on the list? I had one advantage. As an LVAD patient I was entitled to 30 days at the top of the list. The coordinator of the patients would determine the best time for me to go to the top. My disadvantage is my age. Once I reach 70 I would no longer be eligible for a heart transplant from this hospital. In my mind this is the top hospital for the procedure.

Why did I have to know all of these actions? All it does is make my family nervous and jumpy. I just hoped they would call and tell them one way or the other. I can live with either.

They did make the call and **I was accepted into the program!!!**

The haze and its effects

Again I am looking into my magic mirror. I can see that the old man with draping skin has a bit of a smile. He is standing a little straighter but is still 40 pounds lighter than the time of the first heart attack. Let me see if I can get this guy serious. I have two years to get a heart or I will be scratched. 70 years old is the limit for this operation. My blood type could be a problem as well as the availability of the heart. The emotional entanglement is that someone has to die for me to live. This is the hardest of all and if all goes well I will have to carry it the rest of my life.

This is tough for me because I have had a great life and can get some more years with staying with the LVAD. I have seen enough people die to never wish for someone to die just so I could live. The attachment to life could put me into a quandary that would allow depression with either choice. It is times like this I just look up and around. I take a deep breath and exhale slowly. I pull in as much nature as I can while saying, "With all of this, and how it fits, how can I not say thank you God!" The higher entity I call my God brings me closer to the rest of the world. You may call God by many different names but all our beliefs end with the same God and in my mind it becomes, "our God!" I will use the word fate so no one is offended. I can now live with my choice because I will rely on fate.

There is one more important factor I must consider. The LVAD is tough on the body and the blood thinners do not help my overall health. I am weak, poor endurance, and I have to be on a certain diet that inhibits weight gain. All of this weighs on me a bit but I can rationalize. The one that I have no way of rationalizing is the pressure on my wife.

She makes herself do everything even though I am more than capable. The hospital has her phone number to call if a heart becomes available. No matter where she is the phone is not far from her hand. If you knew my wife this is almost normal except for the pressure of hurry up and wait. The meals are planned around my diet. She calls every time I am scheduled to take a medicine. My wife is fulfilling the saying, "It is the care giver that takes the beating."

Hedging your bets

The heart transplant team had faith in their skills and in me. They wanted me to live at least until the chances of getting a heart were made available to me. The team scheduled me for a procedure to have a pacemaker with a defibrillator put into my chest. I was told that in case a heart becomes available they would like me to be alive.

It took all my patience to have the procedure. I was told one day but it turned into two days in a hospital room. The nurse came into the room while I was waiting for the doctor to see if I was going to be discharged. She explained that I would be leaving in a while. I laid there for a minute and smiled as I began to take off all the monitoring contacts on my body. The nurse came in the room and with quick breath explained that I cannot take them off until the discharge papers are delivered. Two steps forward and one back! Again.

Just the beginning

I could not dwell on the heart transplant. I had to use a mindset that the LVAD was the destination. In my area there are only two cardiac rehabilitation classes. Each resided in a hospital. I chose one and began the rehabilitation of the body. There were about six of us in the class. The room was equipped with specialized machines, dumb bells, treadmills, and stationary cycles. A program was written by the nurse and we began the exercising.

When you get to the place you are required to wear a monitor. You put the electrodes on yourself which are in turn hooked into the monitor. The readings that are monitored resemble an EKG I would get on my visits to the hospital. They won't let my heart rate go beyond 97 on any of my exercises. I would drive myself there three times a week and enjoy the pain and pressure knowing that my future may depend on what I am doing now. Every time I would enter the garage at the hospital I would say out loud. It is only the **beginning** of the time I have left.

Let's pump up the pressure

We finally have a routine. The times of medication and meals has stabilized. I walk and go to rehabilitation. It is now I begin to think of work. My world is divided into few things but one of the entries is work. I rode to the college to talk to my boss and fellow educators. I needed to see a reaction from them and hear their tones as we talked to understand that with an LVAD do they believe I can teach successfully. My first impression was not as positive as I had wanted. At home I again looked into a mirror and began to see the drawn face of the old man. My magic mirror hid this from me.

I walked longer and at rehab I worked harder. In the middle of the night I worked my feet twice the amount of time. I was almost at the point in my development that I would ask about teaching a class. It was then that a phone call was received. For the next thirty days I was being put at the top of the A list. I was waiting for a

heart in the largest section of the country. The
heart had to be a specific blood type. I am a little
older and if I don't get a heart in these thirty days
the chance of not getting one becomes greater. I
think you understand it is now the term fate
becomes important. The term fate keeps me
from praying for a heart that must come from a
person who is dead or dying. In my mind prayer
should never be used in a negative direction. It
is the power of prayer that I am here at all.
Again it was not me but my family the pressure
was applied. Pressure that they had no control to
change.

I feel for them. The pressure of feelings is the
worst. They spent a great deal of time waiting to
see if I would die or live. More waiting is the
menu. They have no choice but to take part.
You have to feel for them as you try to
understand the situation yourself. I still meditate
but I am not as good as I used to be in my youth.
It still helps me focus and understand the only
view or reaction that I can evaluate or control.
That is mine.

I have had a marvelous life and on the day it
ends it will be too soon. But it will be a day
filled with contentment and satisfaction. That is

why I feel for them. I am fine with the next step. I haven't written it down yet but the philosophy of the New Orleans funeral is the way I wish to go out. The sad movement of the blues is played and marched to as you go to the cemetery. We are all a bit sad when someone we know dies. I have seen a number of my friends buried but a little while later you remember them a little younger, funnier, and with their good qualities. You smile and they will never grow older or leave you as long as you can sit under that tree and dream.

It is important to remember that in New Orleans the music is festive, the dancing is done with a smile, a laugh, and a lightness of step. This is how they leave the cemetery and celebrate the life of the person they just buried.

I am still striving for status quo

I weighed approximately 195 pounds on the day of my first heart attack. After a few stays at hospitals I left the last one with an LVAD and about 150 pounds. I have been trying to put weight on but on my present diet, medication, and blood thinners it is a bit difficult. The optimism is in full gear. I believe that I will be teaching even with the LVAD. My weight has stabilized and is increasing as my rehabilitation is progressing to a good destination. I promised my wife that I would carry the cane for one year and I am trying to keep my promise. I literally carry the cane most times trying to walk properly with no lean. Yes, Things are beginning to take shape and life will be steady and understood. When I was a younger I would do things on a whim and think of the results later. I gathered a lot of memories with that philosophy. I only had one rule. Never do anything that would hurt someone else. When I married and had children I needed routine. It helped with my division between work and family. I worked a lot. But now it was all coming together. Then the phone call.

Chaos and the hope of organization

I was sitting downstairs when the phone rang. All these months and I don't think my wife was more than 3 inches from her phone at any time. She came to the steps and said it was for me. It was the hospital saying that they have procured a heart and I am to come into the hospital. I was already packed as they suggested. We only had to pick up the case and go. When we got there

we were asked was this our first time. This is
when we found out that even after all the
preparation I may not get the transplant. This
hospital is one of the top heart transplant hospital
in the country. One reason is they send their
own doctors to do the cursory examination of the
heart. If it passes their initial examination then
we end up where I currently am. If for some
reason on the closer exam something is wrong
they would send me home. From this point I
only know they prepped me for the operation and
wheeled me into the room. This was about five
hours after I checked into the suite.

From this point I can only write about what I
was told and the answers to my questions. The
heart was in good condition and I was the first to
be operated. I say the first because there were a
number of other operating rooms being utilized.
The lead team handled my heart transplant with
the follow up team doing all the closing
procedures. I found out later following me were
two lung transplants, one kidney, and a liver. I
had a chance to meet and talk to some of these
people while recuperating. Each one gave me
the emotional response of a new individual
seeing life for the first time. Each one I was able

to talk with had the same response I did.
Someone had to die for us to have the new view
of life. I will think of this more now than I did
before the transplant. But for now, this day,
death takes a holiday.

After my operation I woke in a large room in
the only bed next to the nurse's station. I was in
one of five rooms with post-operative patients. I
raised the bed so I could view my body. I had
five hoses in my body with each draining into a
bucket on the floor. Apparently I went into the
operation at 191 pounds and came out at about
220. It is like planting a plant, bush, or tree.
Soak it with water to minimize the shock to the
organic. The hoses entering the body were not
sutured. I was bed bound until the hoses drained
most of the fluids.

Did everything go as planned? Sometimes
you have to improvise. I found out that when
they were removing the LVAD there was a small
problem. A tear occurred in the artery. I have
always admired a doctor or anyone that could do
a good job at what they were doing. In this case
I am thankful that one of doctors had a large
thumb. He or she put the thumb to work and
plugged the dike. Again luck was with me.

Everything seemed to go well. That little expression is always followed by oops!

Tubes, drains, and hope

The tubes in the chest were just about done so the hoses had to come out. The surgeon came in to do it and take a little pride in his work. Each doctor I dealt with in this hospital had a swagger to their step and pride in their work. As a patient I love to see this. He only had trouble with one hose that was beginning to attach itself. The cure? Pull real hard!! I had a small problem called deep vein thrombosis. Once that was stabilized it was found that the heart was very healthy except it came with a yeast infection. Apparently this is a problem. Since they don't know where to put the cream I needed a strong antibiotic delivered intravenous in the hospital. They put a pick line in after collapsed veins became a problem. The antibiotic has a few side effects but only one that concerned me. I was told it hardly ever happens. You could go blind!

Here I lie with the chest tubes out and an intravenous antibiotic dripping into my body. Now I can start looking forward. You need a base to move forward and this cannot get any

wilder. The doctors were coming around and
they came in to see me. The one pocket above
my left leg was not draining properly. As they
tell me something they always pause. I think it
is the point I am to panic or ask questions. They
looked – I looked – and then they told me. They
would like to do something called a lap. They
would cut my muscle at the top of the thigh and
move it over the pocket to allow it to dry. The
plastic surgery team would do this and there
would be no problem with the procedure. I
followed my philosophy of, if I give control to
the doctors then my answer is yes as long as I am
in the hospital.

The doctor came in and said I was now
stabilized and I could be discharged. I looked at
the tube in my arm and he said that would go
with me. I had previously talked to the doctor in
charge of infectious diseases and he said there
was a pill of the liquid going into me that could
work. No one wanted it but I left without the
intravenous tubes. In place of those tubes I had a
cane, pills and two tubes coming out of my
thigh. The tubes were each about 18 inches
ending in a bulb. They were draining the liquid
so the top of the leg could dry. I would empty

each every night and record the fluid drained. Each could be concealed under my pants.

It may not have looked it but I now had the beginning I needed to work myself into shape. I need to be as fit as possible for my wife and family. I owe it to the young person who died and in turn I got a new heart. I need to settle in physically and mentally for the rest of my life. I can do this because it is who I am! If you say it enough maybe you will believe it.

The veil on the mirror is lifted

A new heart and a schedule of visits to the hospital to check on my condition. It was explained to me that I could expect to come in every two weeks for a biopsy and blood tests. The progression would be every two weeks, once a month, once every three months, once every six months, and once a year. The schedule would take about three to four years.

I began the visits and eventually didn't need the leg tubes. I was walking a lot and thought it was about time to see if I would be accepted at the college. I was anxious to get into the classroom to do something productive. I think it was a way of saying I want to be somewhere that

other people would treat me as if I was normal
and wouldn't break if I exerted myself. I went
and saw my boss. She is a woman of integrity
and purpose who I respect. I asked about
teaching in the fall and she was agreeable with
the idea. The world was beginning to take shape.
I almost have a bounce to the step.

I first had to see if I had the stamina to teach.
I would go downstairs and turn on the television.
I would watch a show or listen to music. It
really did not matter. Whatever it was I would
do it standing upright. I would stand and move
to a designated spot as if I were in a classroom. I
would do this for two and one half hours. This
would be done once every night that no one was
home.

The time has come. I have a class and I am
ready to go. Wow! I can still tie a tie. I will be
there early as I have been for every job I have
ever had. In the classroom I stand alone walking
the probable path I will use for the lecture. Let
me take stock of where I am at the moment. I
can walk slow and will look as if I have good
balance. I use the cane a little but attempt to
stand straight. I have a nice scar going down my
chest where the zipper was located. Zipper

means the staples used to close me. I have very little feeling on the top of my feet but they seem to be getting better. There is no feeling on the top of my left thigh. The little finger on my right hand tingles and does not have full feeling. This will affect my writing on the board but I have spent the last twenty minutes practicing. My stamina is still short but when pushed I can do this. Let's hope I am correct. I am sitting now and the first student enters the room. I had my first heart attack on September 3, 2014. I am sitting watching a student enter and it is September 2, 2015. The one day means I did not complete the year and I can now look to the possibilities of the future. How something so simple can mean so much is amazing! **The veil has been removed!!**

A disease and no child in sight

I made it through the semester. I am on top of the world. The holidays have come and gone. The family is healthy and I am a bit more generous than before my heart attacks. There may be something to the story of Scrooge. The reserve in the bank is a little lower and I am a little lighter of foot. I look around and can only smile. The order in my life is finally returning.

The slight smile has returned. I have my class set for the spring semester.

But there is that saying, "Things happen". It is like you just paid your car off and the transmission needs work. My appetite lessened and my stamina decreased. My wife noticed this and said we should see a doctor. With my infinite wisdom I said no and just tried to eat more and push my endurance. I just didn't want to stay overnight in a hospital room. My wife did what any mother would do for her 5 year old child. She made a quick appointment and I was now in the doctor's office at the hospital. They must know me because the doctor that came in was, "**The Doctor**".

He looked at me and said that I had to stay for a while. It happens the transplant was from a person who had a virus called CMV. If you have ever had a fever blister than you know the virus. This is a member of the herpes family and most children on the east coast have it by the age of eight. The problem is I was raised on the west coast and elsewhere. It is not as prevalent. I can no longer say I have never had it. This would require a hospital stay and intravenous medicine. The same medicine I took for the yeast infection.

I didn't teach my spring class. The thought of
the stay coupled with the medicine must have
been tough on me because my blood pressure
increased. Part of my medication now included
blood pressure pills. I agreed to this with the
understanding that when I leave the hospital the
blood pressure pills stay.

My wife would visit every day and I had a
good nurse. He is one of the few nurses that
actually read my file. All the nurses liked me
because I would shut my door and not ask for
anything. They would see me when they had to
check on me or one of the four times I would
walk the halls. I would carry my cane and
everyone in a white coat would tell me that is not
how to use a cane. I would have to explain that I
promised my wife I would carry it for one year.
They had trouble locating the virus but after a
week they said I could go home. It is here that
the child in me comes to the forefront.

I explained that I will stay as long as you
wish but I do not go home with a pick line.
There was a young doctor who did everything in
her power to get me to go home with the pick
line and blood pressure medicine. She was a
little on the dark side for just a bit when she told

me the worst effects it would have if I didn't go home with it. I tried once to explain that while in the hospital my veins collapse. One of my sons had a lot of problems when he came home with one. She even wrote in my discharge papers that I could possibly suffer traumatic effects. I went home with pills.

The blood pressure pills I would not take home. I explained that for the last 5 months minimum I have been taking my blood pressure twice a day. The average was in the range of 122/82. I also explained the new survey that I read. Blood pressure increase was measured when a person is in the doctor's office. This became known as white coat syndrome. A doctor cannot make a diagnosis on 4 to 10 readings in a year. It is not reliable and the patient will be on the medication the rest of their life. I have been in studies while in college dealing with blood pressure readings. I even played with changing the pressure while sitting, standing, and crossing the legs. I promised to monitor my pressure and if the increase persisted then I would notify the heart team. So far I have been within safe limits.

Never give up trying to be normal … for me

Well, here we go again. I look, smile, and laugh a bit out loud. My magic mirror did not reply. It just showed me a man that was tired and looked like he could use a pick me up of some type. Time for the analysis. The CMV seemed to knock out progress in some of the areas I have been trying to improve. Feeling on the top of my feet was returning a little as well as the feeling in my little finger on my right hand. Feeling is now gone. My left thigh seems to have a harder feel when I lean against it and the area of no feeling has increased. My stamina has decreased and I am out of breath sooner than I would expect. I again look like skin hanging from bones but not as bad as before. This is a practice of mine. Psychology implies a person can look into a mirror and see everything that he believes is wrong. But he will find something good before he leaves the reflection. I am now doing my self-pity party. I have done this many times in the past. Why can't I just wallow and let the world go on its way? It was not the way I was raised. The 5 minutes an adult can give a child. My parents always gave it and we knew to listen without talking. Think of those that are less fortunate then you. By that statement they meant the people who suffered, agonized, and survived.

I had a small list of people that I would think about in these situations. These are a few I have experienced and can feel as if it happened to me. Their problems always made mine seem so small. A young girl of fifteen who glowed from the inside showing innocence, honesty, and empathy for all lost her mother in a car-truck accident. Her father, who was a blue collar genius, became an invalid. The elderly black lady with new knees enduring pain with a simple smile. The prosthetic patients learning how to walk and/or pick up an object. The shouts of pain and bewilderment I would hear in the hospital as I walked the halls. The forgotten veteran who was in the emergency ward at the naval hospital. He was brought in from the streets. An alcoholic suffering the DTs and needing four people to hold down a man of 150 pounds. I now have to add a young person who died leaving a family in turmoil and an old man with a new heart. How can you not try to pull yourself out of self-pity and strive for a normal life? **You owe so many people!**

How many times do you start over?

I have spent many tedious moments as the new kid on the block. A new school with new people. You learned how to observe and not do anything unusual until you knew the hierarchy. If there was a disagreement it should be with one of the top dogs and not someone lower. That would mean that you would have to work your way up the ladder. I have started over many times and just thought it was natural. This time it seemed different. This new start could set the tone for the rest of my life. Time is relative. As I write this I know I have been granted an extension. The length of this extension could be a midsummers dream or last a couple of decades. My work ethic, a lot of luck, and the breath of God will be needed as I find my new life. You have often heard the expression that today is the first day of the rest of your life. For me the expression has a stronger meaning then when I used to say it to myself many mornings.

What life can I expect?

Physically I am weak. I will be needing an exercise schedule and the mental strength to do it consistently. That is the part I can do because its success depends on my will power. There is one part of the rest of my life that concerns me. It is my memory. When I woke from the coma I was told I lost some long term memory as well as some short term memory. They did not tell me right away and did not sit with me face to face to tell me what I could expect. It seems I am on a journey. The quality of life in front of me depends on my will, determination, and knowing the limits of my memory. Let me first work the physical. This is more quantitative and something I understand.

As the snow falls it gives you a clean look

January 9, 2017. This is the day of my visit to the hospital. Every three months I go to the hospital for extensive blood tests and a biopsy. The blood tests are important because I am on three medications that are called lifesaving medicines. Two of these medicines reduce my immune system to keep rejection of the heart low enough that the body can utilize it without stress. The third is a medication that helps protect my kidneys from the other two medications. I currently take nine pills in the morning and five pills in the evening. Most of the other pills are vitamins and supplements that the doctors wish me to take. Most of the medications can be bought over the counter at the local drugstore.

It is Saturday before my hospital visit and it is snowing lightly. It has already covered the ground with a thin cover of the white blanket you see on the Christmas cards. As I look outside my fireplace is on and I evaluate my present situation. My physical status is very important to me. It has been over two years since my coma. During the coma I lost almost all my muscle integrity and structure. The atrophy was terrible. There was not much I could do with the LVAD for almost a year and then the advent of CMV. The CMV put me into the hospital for a while. I had been exercising at home recently with some dumbbells. My thoughtful older brother gave be some money and said this should cover a gym. On December 29 I did my first visit and workout at the gym. I wrote the schedule of exercises and have been doing them three times a week until my next semester begins. The following are the exercises and initial weights used. They are all machine oriented as was my cardiac rehab after the LVAD. This is important for body orientation while the exercise is being done.

Workout Schedule of exercises and weights used

Exercise	Weight/setting
Warmup(treadmill)	3.5
AB crunch	60 lbs
Lateral raise	30 lbs
Shoulder press	20 lbs
Triceps press	50 lbs
Triceps extension	30 lbs
Biceps curl	30 lbs
Hammer crunch	10 lbs
Treadmill	3.5/4.0
Pectoral fly	25 lbs
Torso rotation	50 lbs
Treadmill	3.5

The body is very important to me. The reason is not that I want to enter a swimsuit contest. It is something that I can see an improvement with and know that I am making progress. The mind is the wall that I must understand and cope with in my everyday situations. People around me, meaning my well intentioned family, treat me as if I can do nothing and will break if I try. I understand that I must tolerate much of this because these people anguished for me while I was struggling in the hospital multiple times. Pride is part of my makeup. No matter the individual, life is appreciated and enjoyed if you have a bit of pride in yourself and those around you. This is shown throughout history and why you do hear the danger. Don't have too much pride that you can't see the truth. I push myself all the time and this bothers people. Those that know me should by this time understand that I always push but never go over my line that would hurt others or me. I know I am still recovering and I am in my 70th year but I am not yet ready to sit in a chair all day.

It has been over two years since my coma and I am just beginning to realize some of the effects. I can see improvement in the physical and that is needed. I have been taught in school at an early age that everyone should have long term goals with the understanding that these may change in time. But it is very important that you have short term goals that can be attained to get there. My short term goal is the physical. I understand it, I can do it, and it can be measured. After the coma I understood that I lost some long term and some short term memory. It is only now that I am understanding the amount of what I lost. This is a hard thing to measure. As I look outside today and see the snow I realize that I have survived and experienced many things that gave me memories that not many people have. And the snow shows me a new and clean beginning can be started at any age. More on the memory after I try to remember some of the frustrations.

Everyone still needs the "A"

When you have a biopsy it is fascinating. You lay on your back and turn your head to the left. The doctor will push a wire through the right side of the neck and it will eventually get to the heart so they can grab a little bit for testing. They need five small pieces from different parts of the heart to see if there is any rejection. They also take blood from the neck for extensive testing. The grades you are interested in come out a few days later and a few days later it is on the computer for me to look and analyze. It is only now that I want to be on the honor roll. As I look at the results I get to sneer with a slight cockiness, because I made the honor roll.

Biopsy and mental therapy ... who knew?

I find the biopsy interesting. Most times they let me look at the screen and see how the wire is progressing in the heart. You also get to see your blood pressure as he is pushing the wire to the heart. With being able to look you have to have complete confidence in the doctor. On the path to the heart the lung could be punctured as well as a few other things. This brings to mind the first biopsy I had. It was shortly after the transplant and I was still in the hospital. I was on the table with my head turned as a young female doctor was being instructed on how to move the wire. This is a teaching hospital. I have a tendency to doze went they don't let me see the screen. I was just relaxing and I could hear from the doctor's lips, "oh, s**t". I chuckled and attempted to relax again. Shortly after this the doctors had a little problem going through the veins, whether it was the left or right side. I do not believe there was any connection. For the next three biopsies I had to go on a different day and check into the hospital. They would knock me out and go from the groin to the heart. I would spend two hours recuperating and go home. It would take the entire day.

It seems that every time I would get a biopsy the doctor would say I was dry and need to hydrate. On the last one I drank two bottles of water before the biopsy and it still was said to me. Next time I will go for three. I am currently at the three month stage for biopsies. At the hospital I would go to a special area with the paper work for the biopsy and test tubes for the blood. The first time I went there as an outpatient there were a number of people in the waiting room. I could only think of the time I will have to spend getting the biopsy and when can I go home. Once the pity party in my head was done I found out all the people getting a biopsy were with transplanted hearts. Almost all of us getting the biopsy were accompanied with a caregiver. My wife would talk with all of them and I would listen. There were few questions that I would ask but all of them would be concerned with their return to a normal way of life.

On the outside you would pay a lot of money for therapy this effective. Almost to a person I was told each was able to return to their previous life in terms of activities and sometimes their job. It seemed they had an inner peace and to that I think I know the answer. They had all figured out what my mother knew. It is all put together in two phrases. **"This too will pass"** and the old favorite **"Everything works out for the best."** With these two phrases and my parent's everyday activities they were able to raise three children who understood patience, compassion, competition, and how to get back up on the horse. Thanks MOM!

Life after death.....Well, almost death

I am approaching my two year anniversary of my heart transplant. The first feeling I always have is the bitter sweet taste of life. I take a deep breath and slowly let it out. A ritual every morning when I leave the house and feel the air of freedom. It is the slow exhale that I remember the young girl who died and in the course of events allowed me to live. The eyes water as I think of the family that still misses her. It is then that I say to myself, "I hope I have and will have lived a life that you would see with pride. Thank You!"

How am I doing? For two years with the new heart and the nine months on the LVAD I have not stopped self-evaluations. I would do this frequently and honestly. Each time I did it I could see an improvement and I would smile. I knew I was ready for life and I was back! Then it would be time for the next evaluation. I would say the same thing. The other thing in my head would be how wrong I was on the last evaluation. The improvements are still coming and I now work harder to keep them coming. It is almost like the endorphins a runner gets when he hits the proverbial wall. In my mind it means that I am ready to live and it only gets better from here.

Three years…..Is there a lesson?

The adventure I have just written was done to the best of my memory. I have missed a lot. I hope I have hit the high points. As I close the abstract I should cover a few topics. The first is a summary of events. This should also highlight the physical and mental roller coaster. The second should mention a couple of pillars that I leaned on. The third should be my hopes and dreams from here to there.

Looking back is ok.......Just don't stare

2013 September I had a heart attack. Within the next two weeks I had two more heart attacks. Each one of the three was major and could have killed me. Each one of the three could have damaged my body and/or mind permanently. During those three weeks I flat lined two times. I was given last rites. My first out of body experience was at the hospital they gave me last rites.

I was hospitalized after the third heart attack and in a short time I was in a coma. The coma began with machines to aid in my life sustaining needs. These machines gave way to life support machines. Ecmo plasma machines were added to run blood through the body while adding gases and probably other medical needs. During the coma they performed three heart oblations and one heart oblation while on ecmo plasma. Heart oblation means to go inside and cut scar tissue away. During the coma I was shocked with paddles at least one or two times a day when my heart rate would be above 200. While in the coma I flat lined four times. A young woman doctor went the extra step and paddled me 27 times during the four flat lines. Her persistence or my stubbornness, I don't know which but I lived. Still in the coma, an LVAD is put into my chest to aid the heart in pumping blood. Then for some reason after approximately two months the eyes opened.

Once awake, a realization of hands and feet paralyzed. The impact of memory loss and the observation of almost no muscle structure. People telling me about the coma said tubes were in every space between my fingers and toes. Tubes from the groin, neck, and stomach could also be seen. Learning how to sit up as well as walking. Tests and more tests as the days went on. A few times the pressure bandage would not hold after the tests and I would bleed, soaking everything around me. Blood thinners were helping me live and the consequence was little compared to the benefit.

I go home with a memory I still test. The body is unproven and the family does not know

how to treat me. I stumble or have to get a glass
and they either do it for me or warn me not to do
something. The way I am treated is much
different than before the heart attacks. For me,
as most people, is appreciated and I can't wait
until it stops. Cardiac rehabilitation is begun. I
can drive and hope to work. I take many tests
and interviews to qualify for a heart transplant. I
qualify and go to the hospital for a new heart.

A new heart and the hope I last long enough
to help the family. I also wish to give the family
of the young person whose heart I just got
satisfaction that did good work with the extra
time. It would give them some consolation that
the heart of their child allowed me the time to
educate many more young minds. Many of these
are future nurses.

I had some immediate problems capped with
a deep vein thrombosis experience. Surgery was
done on my leg to cut a muscle and move it to
improve the healing process.

I was trying to understand my current
situation and a doctor walks in and says I have a
yeast infection. I barely understand that concept
with a woman. Intravenous medicine with the

byproduct of possible blindness. This was
followed by CMV. A childhood ailment that
knocked me on my tail.

Two year anniversary has just past. My
weight has stabilized and my energy is good.
My stamina is improving. I am at the stage that
when I hurt or need to slow down I can't just say
it was my hospital adventure. It could be that I
am just an old fart.

An odd assortment of people......I call them family

In everyday life you meet a number of people.
My brothers and I view people in a simplified
matter. People that show attributes repugnant to
us are people we only meet once. This concept
has kept us from frustration with people we
could only call acquaintances. Family on the
other hand cannot have a rating attached since
you do not have the option of only meeting them
once. I must say that all the family members
gave the support that was needed. My wife and
her sisters, my two brothers, and my sons gave
as much as was needed. Caregivers always take
a beating. It was good to see so many share the

burden. I could not have done much without my wife.

I cannot say too much about the family that worried about me. I imagine a person having to put down a dog that has been like a family member. I have been in that situation and knew I was doing right by the dog but the sense of loss was great. My family faced my death more than one time and the emotional toll is something I can never take away from them. I can only lean on the expression, **"you do what is needed for family."**

There is much of the past I cannot remember…The future looks great!

My sons have gone their own way in the world and each has a fine wife to share their futures. I know their problems will be many and with each problem that is solved their union and family will become unique and stronger.

One of my pleasures in life were the times I could people watch. I would see the strength and patience they would try to use. Many were successful. I hope to see my sons and their families not just survive in this tough world but to grow and enjoy those around them. My time left is like everyone else's. It is unknown but the end will not be feared. I have an advantage that many people don't. All the time from when I awoke from the coma is extra. It is a dream that became truth. A wish that has been with me since I was a pup. The wish was not for happiness but for contentment. What a feeling to know I lived, died, and was content with the life I lived. I now am living on the extension. The offer I should make to the higher plane essence, the one we all call by different names, the one with no name cannot be sufficient. I owe so much for my life I have lived. The reality of truth is all I have. I close my eyes and feel the music of contentment and I can only say thank you, **"God!"**

Epilogue

As I grew I had many goals. I wanted to go through life and never hurt anyone. Take the late sixties away and I have almost accomplished it. Another goal was to continue from early childhood the idea of never making fun of another individual. My parents were convinced that the hurt on the inside is much harder to heal than the hurt on the outside. I can say that I am doing well. I do remember a time when I didn't say anything when friends of mine made fun of another person in a hurtful manner. I was in sixth grade.

When I was old enough I began collecting memories. I did many different activities and went to many places while I was growing. I realized then that at an older age I could sit back and remember a time when. I had a long list of events that I could bring back just with a thought and the smile would be slight. The warmth I would feel would last a long time.

The loss of some short and long term memory hurts. There are years I cannot bring back. There are names of people I worked with for years that I don't immediately remember. I see a

term and I have to write it down so I don't
immediately forget it. I am lecturing to a class
for two to four hours and I have to use sentences
that have words I know I will not forget. Yes, it
hurts. Whether it comes back some or stays
blank is not known.

My attitude has always been a wonder to me.
How did I grow looking at the bright side of life?
How is it that I and my two brothers have never
argued or fought? We are always there for each
other. Why do we know our religion and some
others and yet never judge another's religion?
My parents. "Wow!." That says it all. How did
they do it? My father from Mississippi and my
mother from Philadelphia. I am currently
writing about this as therapy and interest.

I am trying to live for those around me
because I owe them. I am attempting to lead a
normal life but there is weight to a new heart as I
remember a young person who died. I think of
my family, who dealt with my death for the
months I was in a coma and all the personnel that
put up with this old man. I have returned to
teaching and at this moment I am entering my
forty eighth year doing the job that I have always
enjoyed. I will pass on as much knowledge as I

can for the length of time they allow me to teach
at the college. I hope that I can show each that
the stress they had and the pain that accompanied
it was worth it.